Cultural Performances

STUDIEN ZUR KULTURPOLITIK
CULTURAL POLICY

Herausgegeben von / Edited by Prof. Dr. Wolfgang Schneider

BAND 21

Zu Qualitätssicherung und Peer Review der vorliegenden Publikation:

Die Qualität der in dieser Reihe erscheinenden Arbeiten wird vor der Publikation durch den Herausgeber der Reihe geprüft.

Notes on the quality assurance and peer review of this publication:

Prior to publication, the quality of the works published in this series is reviewed by the editor of the series.

Shadrach Teryila Ukuma

Cultural Performances

A Study on Managing Collective Trauma amongst
Displaced Persons in Daudu, Benue State, Nigeria

PETER LANG

Bibliographic Information published by the Deutsche Nationalbibliothek
The Deutsche Nationalbibliothek lists this publication in the Deutsche
Nationalbibliografie; detailed bibliographic data is available online at
http://dnb.d-nb.de.

Library of Congress Cataloging-in-Publication Data
A CIP catalog record for this book has been applied for at the
Library of Congress.

Zugl.: Hildesheim, Univ., Diss., 2020

Hil 2
ISSN 1611-700X
ISBN 978-3-631-83953-9 (Print)
E-ISBN 978-3-631-83954-6 (E-PDF)
E-ISBN 978-3-631-83955-3 (EPUB)
E-ISBN 978-3-631-83956-0 (MOBI)
DOI 10.3726/b17754

© Peter Lang GmbH
Internationaler Verlag der Wissenschaften
Berlin 2021
All rights reserved.

Peter Lang – Berlin · Bern · Bruxelles · New York · Oxford · Warszawa · Wien

This publication has been peer reviewed.

www.peterlang.com

Dedication

To all victims of violent conflicts battling trauma issues, especially those of the farmers/herders conflict in Benue State, whose unfortunate circumstances became for me the inspiration and material for this research.

Acknowledgements

This research was possible because of several reasons. God in His infinite mercies made it possible for me to be part of the golden opportunity made available through the DAAD funded SDG Graduate School "Performing Sustainability: Cultures and Development in West Africa". I appreciate the partner institutions which include the Universities of Hildesheim (Germany), Maiduguri (Nigeria), and Cape Coast (Ghana), as led by Prof. Dr. Raimund Vogels, Prof. Abba I. Tijani and Prof. Florian Carl.

I owe a huge debt of gratitude to my supervisors, Prof. Sunday Enessi Ododo, Prof. Dr. Wolfgang Schneider, and Prof. Haruna D. Dlakwa, for their support, tutelage, and patience. Sirs, you offered me a level of friendship and camaraderie that has now grown beyond student-teacher levels. I am eternally grateful for this.

My gratitude also goes to the Coordinators of the SDG Graduate School in the partner Universities. They include Drs. Chris Mtaku (Nigeria), Eyram Fiagbedzi (Ghana), Nepomuk Riva and Meike Lettau (Germany).

Especial thanks to my wife Nelly Mnena Ukuma, who endured three long years of my absence, short attention, half affection, and impatience. You are a strong woman, my everyday choice and I love you! My parents built in me the zeal for education and service. My father, Simon Asongo Ukuma has a profound belief in me which gives me the audacity to face life challenges without looking back. I thank you Sir. I believe my mum Doo Ann Ukuma (nee Mnger) will be looking down from heaven with satisfaction; fond memories of her are a ball of energy for me always. I love you both endlessly.

Prof. Tor Iorapuu had special interest in my research and offered useful insights. He gave me books and created time to discuss my research questions. Prof. Gowon Ama Doki saw the academic promise in me and helped set before me a clear path for my academic career. Rev. Brother Moses Abunya, fsc, PhD, bought five books important to this research from the United States and shipped to me. Mr. Nathaniel Msen Awuapila has mentored me in many ways. I thank them both immeasurably.

Several friends have been nice to me and I will mention a few:Rev. Fr. Solomon Mfa, Drs. Elijah Terdoo Ikpanor, and Zack Wade, Moses Kamnan, Festus Mbapuun, Isaac Akaa, Binwie Tanwie, Samuel Ude, Vitalis Kpev, Ayande Timothy, and Benjamin Igbo.

Lastly, but most importantly, I appreciate the scholarly endeavours of authors whose works I generously helped myself with in developing my own ideas. Thank you all!

Shadrach Teryila Ukuma
Makurdi, Nigeria
June 5, 2020

Contents

Dedication 5

Acknowledgements 7

List of Figures 13

List of Plates 15

Foreword 17

Introduction 21

1 Cultural Performances, Collective Trauma Management
   and the Farmer/Herder Conflicts: An Introduction 25

   1.1 Statement, Objectives and Questions of the Study 28

   1.2 The Farmers/Herders Conflicts in Benue 31

       1.2.1 Triggers and Enablers to the Conflict in the Benue Valley 34

       Climate Change 34

       Depleting Space for Farming 34

       Corruption 34

       Lack of Political Will 35

       1.2.2 Government's Response to the Farmers/Herders' Conflict 36

       1.2.3 Efforts by Civil Society Organizations 38

2 Conceptualisations and Theories 39

   2.1 Conceptual Orientation 39

       2.1.1 Cultural Performance 39

2.1.2 Cultural Sustainability 41

Procedural Sustainability 43

2.1.3 Collective Trauma 45

2.1.4 Community Building 50

2.2 Indigenous African Performances and Cultural Reflectivity 55

2.3 Performance, Culture and the Building of Sustainable
Communities 60

2.4 Therapeutic Performance and Performance Therapy 61

Music Therapy 63

Dance/Movement Therapy 66

Drama Therapy 68

2.5 Collective Trauma and Collective Healing 71

2.6 Nigeria's Cultural Policy, the Arts and Culture in Social
Transformation 74

2.7 Theories 77

2.7.1 Cultural Performance Theory 78

Liminality 79

Reflexivity 82

2.7.2 Social Practice Theory 86

2.8 Conclusion 87

3 Methodology 89

3.1 Research Design 89

3.2 Study Population and Sample 90

3.3 Data Collection Methods 91

3.4 Procedure for Data Collection 91

3.5 Method of Data Analysis 92

3.6 Validity and Reliability 92

3.6.1 Multiple Data Collection Methods 93

3.6.2 Member-Checks 93

3.7 Ethical Considerations 94

3.7.1 Participant Language 94

3.7.2 Informed Consent 94

3.8 Data Management 95

3.9 Researcher Positionality 95

3.10 Conclusion 96

4 The Cultural Performances 97

4.1 Cultural Performances amongst the Tiv 97

4.2 Cultural Performances by the Displaced Persons in Daudu
Community 102

4.2.1 Music: Folk Songs 105

4.2.2 Dance and Movement 112

4.2.3 Dramatic Enactments 113

4.3 Contextual Findings 117

4.3.1 Functions of Cultural Performances in Daudu Community 119

4.3.1.1 Identity: 119

4.3.2 Extent of Knowledge on the Effect of Cultural
Performances in Managing Collective Trauma in Victims
of Violent Conflicts 121

4.3.3 Applying Cultural Performances in Managing Collective
Trauma 122

4.3.4 Challenges of Cultural Performances in Managing
Collective Trauma 125

4.3.5 Strategies for Effective Use of Cultural Performances in
Managing Collective Trauma 128

4.4 Findings from Systematic Review of Literature 130

4.5 Conclusion 135

5 Managing Collective Trauma 137

5.1 Findings 137

5.1.1   Cultural Performances Help in Managing Collective Trauma 137

5.1.2   Subjective Dispositions Affect Extent of Effect 138

5.1.3   Communal Lifestyle of Victims Is an Asset 139

5.1.4   Women and Children Are More Open to Using Cultural
Performances to Engage Their Trauma 140

5.1.5   Escapism is Crucial 140

5.1.6   Improvisation and Spontaneity as Key Elements 141

5.1.7   Community Building in Performance 142

5.2   A Cultural Performance Model for Managing Collective Trauma 143

5.3   The Daudu Experience and Transformation of Farmers/Herders
Conflicts 145

5.4   The Cultural Sustainability and Community Building Implication .. 146

5.5   The Cultural Policy Imperative 149

5.6   Conclusion 151

6   Cultural Performances, Collective Trauma Management,
Cultural Sustainability and Policy: Conclusion and
Outlook 153

6.1   Summary 153

6.2   Conclusion 155

6.3   Contribution to Knowledge 156

6.4   Limitations of Study 158

6.5   Suggestions for Further Research 158

6.6   Recommendations 159

References 161

List of Figures

Figure   **Page**

Fig. 1: The Ukuma Illustration on Interconnectivity of African Dance,
        Drama and Music 105

Fig. 2: Ukuma Model for Cultural Performances in Managing
        Collective Trauma 144

List of Plates

Plate   **Page**

Plate 1: Displaced Women at a Singing session (Ukuma 2018) 107

Plate 2: The displaced persons pictured here dancing. The bending posture here communicates how they duck from the weapons of their assailants (Ukuma 2018) 109

Plate 3: A woman is pictured here carrying a child to safety (Ukuma 2018) 110

Plate 4: Researcher joined in the slow and sombre dance (Ukuma 2017) ... 113

Plate 5: Displaced persons dramatizing how they fled with their belongings (Ukuma 2018, UNHCR Shelter, Daudu) 115

Plate 6: Here, a woman falls with her luggage and another assists her (Ukuma 2018, UNHCR Shelter, Daudu) 115

Plate 7: In this scene, the woman in motion is the supposed woman who dropped her baby as she fled. Notice the man in blue behind her picking up the child (Ukuma 2018, UNHCR Shelter, Daudu) 116

Plate 8: Notice here a man trying to help a woman with her child so she could run faster. Another woman bears the burden of a baby and luggage. All these are spontaneous re-enactments of their experiences (Ukuma 2018, UNHCR Shelter, Daudu) 116

Plate 9: Pictured here is a woman rendering the lines in above excerpt. Notice another woman behind sneaking to safety with a child (Ukuma, St. Francis Mission, Daudu, 14/09/2017) 117

Plate 10: Here the woman on the left bends to take aim at a fleeing resident as the attacker would (Ukuma2018, UNHCR Shelter, Daudu) 118

Plate 11: In this scene, a woman falls to the ground as she makes to run, this according to her was what actually happened and she dislocated her ankle in the actual experience. Another woman opens her arms in wait of a child running towards her (Fieldwork, St. Francis Mission, Daudu, 14/09/2017) 118

Foreword

This book *Cultural Performances: A Study on Managing Collective Trauma amongst Displaced Persons in Daudu Community of Benue State, Nigeria* is the outcome of a doctoral thesis. The work examines the performative experiences of victims of violent conflicts between farmers and herders in Nigeria. We are exposed to how these victims, who have been suffering collective trauma, resorted to using cultural performances namely dance, music and dramatic enactments to enhance their well-being and rekindle hope for the future. The Background of this Study reveals that the history of post-independent Nigeria has been awash with series of conflicts, crises and violence with varying underlying causes from one geo-political zone to the other, but the work focuses on the violent conflicts between Herders and Farmers in the Central part of Nigeria, especially Benue State which is one of the worse hit states in Central Nigeria since the return of civil rule in 1999. These occurring conflicts have accounted for the displacement of several communities with critical attendant consequences. Daudu is one of the communities in Guma Local Government Area of Benue State that is so affected. Of serious concern are the living conditions of the displaced persons in Daudu in addition to their memories of the carnage they experienced which account for the collective trauma they suffer. However, in an attempt to cope with the traumatic experiences, they thus resorted to the use of cultural performances as a way of coping and reinventing meaning in their lives.

The work sees cultural performance as an umbrella term encapsulating a wide variety of performance genres evident in a people's daily events and embedded as their way of life. These performances could be those events in which a culture's values are displayed for their perpetuation: rituals such as parades, religious ceremonies, and community festivals as well as conversational storytelling, performances of social and professional roles, and individual performances of race, gender, sexuality, and class. In this way, cultural performances become veritable instruments with which a people move through the world as individuals, construct identity, and build community together. The fundamental aesthetics of cultural performances serves a bifurcated function; one is reflective, i.e. showing ourselves to ourselves, and the second is reflexive, which is arousing consciousness of ourselves to see ourselves. It is in this quintessential role of "showing ourselves to ourselves" and in the aroused consciousness to see ourselves that cultural performances become significant and critical mechanisms for managing collective trauma which is either occasioned by violent conflicts or disasters.

Shadrach Teryila Ukuma further foregrounds the importance of performances, especially their potential and capability to tap into our expressive
aspects of body, mind, and spirit through the use of music, sound, imagery, role
play, dance, and movement. It is noteworthy too that the performative, beyond
its entertainment value, portrays a spectacular representation of a culture, and
it is a mirror for entire societies, where individuals gain an understanding of
themselves in society, and therefore, in life. This means that the performing arts,
and of course cultural performances can be viewed as an expression of a culture's
emotional state while also providing a conglomerate of forms that are all artistic with emotional outlets, creating a symphony of emotions, a wealth of cultural information from the past, as revealed through dramaturgical enactments.
Through the performative, there is created an emotional bond, known as empathy, developed between the performers and the audience. In this way, one can
see that the performing arts do not only heal, but also reflect societal sentiments
within that healing process.

Critical to this study is the farmers/herders conflict that is characterized by
mass atrocities including brutal killings, rape, displacements, destruction of
livelihoods and heritage. It observes that trauma management services remain
in huge deficit in response to the conflict even as there are no medical trauma
specialists attending to the psychoanalytical needs of the victims especially in
the area under study – Daudu. Despite the several strategies adopted by stakeholders to sustain peace in the region, art-based approaches have received little
or no attention.

Cultural Performance theory conceptualizes culture as the centre of hegemonic, or dominating, messages and revealing the hierarchical structure of
society through lived experience. This places culture as the current running
through all of human activity in the various spheres of life. The relationship of
culture and performance is therefore that of a coexisting entity, mutually complimenting each other, and not a means to an end. In this work Cultural performance theory is adopted as a radical tool to identify the root issue, the binary
opposition between theory and practice by providing a model of communicative
practice in which culture and performance are inextricably joined and integral
to the communal experience of everyday life.

Social Practice Theory essentially deals with why people do what they do, and
offers alternative explanations of human 'action' other than behavioural understandings. This in recent time has also been found useful in the study of health
and well-being; it clarifies and acknowledges the materiality of spaces, places and
things in everyday life, and the understandings of how through performance and
the incorporation of new elements into practice, daily routines may change over

time. In this study, the social practice theory is applied to anchor discussions that pertain to performance as a mechanism for managing collective trauma, and performance as a facilitator of cultural sustainability. The argument is that it is from continual practice that aspects of culture or everyday life find the guarantee that they may be relevant in the context of the future. Overall, the thrust of the thesis is that – Cultural performances are important in managing the collective trauma experiences of victims of violent conflicts as they help victims to attain catharsis, build and intense community spirit, deepen resilience and envision a brighter future.

The core of this study centres on the utilitarian potency of Cultural Perfor-mances in managing collective trauma in victims of violent conflicts. Using the displaced persons in Daudu community of Benue State, Nigeria, the researcher demonstrates convincingly robust knowledge of cultural performances of the people especially their music, dance and drama. These are systematically assem-bled and integrated to flesh out how sustainability is embodied and performed from an African cultural context. Cultural sustainability is projected in the study as an emergent property, social practice theory, the embodiment paradigm, and performance theory to justify its acceptance of multiple partial knowledge and the essential need to connect theory with lived reality so that sustainable performances can take centre stage. The study itself is confidently founded on robust and relevant literature that opens up our minds to the inadequacies of Western dominated thoughts on creative art therapies which profiles profession-alism in this area without paying attention to non-Western approaches; indeed the thesis confronts us with other possibilities not reflected in the Western liter-ature. Shadrach Ukuma amply demonstrates scholarly grasp of the field of Cul-tural Sustainability and the strategies for effective use of Cultural Performances in Managing Collective Trauma.

Significantly, this work creates an understanding of how victims of farmers/ herders conflicts deal with their traumatic experiences through cultural perfor-mances in time and space, especially how they negotiate meaning out of their experiences and generate a positive outlook which is needed for their collective well-being and balance in order to lead normal lives. This will consequently lead them to become more disposed towards conflict resolution processes. Also, the work provides empirical evidence for Government agencies and civil society or-ganizations involved in psycho-social support of victims to support their activi-ties, particularly in adopting cultural performances which are the idioms of the people with which they connect easily. Further still, Ukuma's work also equips us with strategies to tame a resurgence of the conflict on the part of the farmers. Through the cultural performance tool, the farmers become less embittered.

With this, Government and civil society organizations will find the basis for policy formulation and implementation in the arts to mainstream cultural performances in the building and deepening of national values such as peaceful coexistence, love and unity in order to attain sustainable development. Finally, researchers will find additional knowledge upon which to build or open up new vistas of scholarly engagements.

It is a stimulant for further research in cultural performances and their therapeutic properties.

Professor S. E. Ododo, fsonta, FNAL
General Manager/Chief Executive
National Theatre, Lagos (Nigeria)
May, 2020

Introduction

By Prof. Dr. Wolfgang Schneider

"Cultural performances are important in managing the collective trauma experiences of victims of violent conflicts as they help victims to attain catharsis, build an intense community spirit, deepen resilience and envision a brighter future". Based on his dissertation as part of the SDG Graduate School "Performing Sustainability: Cultures and Development in West Africa" supported by DAAD, Shadrach's thesis formulates the field of research, the epistemological interest and the research subject to be observed, analysed and deliberated.

He is concerned with the conflicts that arise between farmers and herdsmen in Nigeria, some of whom cultivate arable land as sedentary farmers, while others move their herds around this agricultural landscape to let them graze. He describes them as brutal conflicts that may involve murder, manslaughter, destruction and displacement. Shadrach talks about the victims on the one hand while highlighting the need for long-term policies to facilitate peaceful coexistence on the other. Traditional forms of cultural performances are a means to an end, based on the participants' many years of experience and their forms of artistic expression. Dance, music and theatre should contribute to communication, awaken understanding and resolve conflicts.

The research work is coherently structured and clearly summarises the academic process in six chapters: First, an introduction provides background information, outlines problems and objectives, asks the research questions and describes the relevance of the study. Chapter 2 looks at the extensive literature on the topic. It deals with Indigenous African Performances, cultural reflectivity, and the building of sustainable communities by arts and culture. It also refers to works that deal specifically with therapeutic theatre and psychotherapeutic creative processes. Shadrach also weighs up the country's cultural policy and looks at theories of social transformation, theatre, and social practice. The short third chapter describes the methodology used and details how he set up the participatory observation and survey of those involved. Chapter 4 focuses on cultural performances, examines the forms and functions of the folk songs, movements and dramatic enactments used by displaced persons, and asks about the challenges and strategies. The fifth chapter focuses on management in coping with collective trauma, lists factors for success, and ventures a cultural policy model for cultural performance. The final chapter summarises the findings, draws a conclusion and even gives recommendations for policy and practice.

Shadrach has an excellent understanding of the topic and is close to – sometimes even in the midst of – the action. Despite this, he understands how to maintain a critical distance. He describes as an observer, analyses as a scientist, and understands the need for reflection before coming to a conclusion. It is clear that this topic is personal to him, indeed it has almost become a part of him. Its importance is clear, its contentiousness is tangible, and the substance of his research is also its quality. As his supervisor, I must admit that I did not initially recognise the importance of this aspect of the dissertation. Shadrach writes: "It is important to state also that the motivation for this was born out of the researcher's everyday encounter with the traumatic experiences of displaced persons and the burning desire to do something about the situation". It was only as time went on that I became aware of the special nature of the relationship between the researcher and the research object. I now have great respect for how the doctoral candidate has walked the tightrope between personal involvement and scientific knowledge.

The discourse is also characterised by an ongoing reflection of this special situation, in the context of a graduate school funded by the global north set against the cultural backdrop of the global south. This is already evident in the literature review: "The discourse on performance therapy and therapeutic performance also presented the dominant Western voice in the creative art therapies, a situation that suppresses or relegates the performative cultural practices in creative healing among non-Western societies. This is quite significant in this study as it directly links to a gap that studying cultural performances as a mechanism for managing collective trauma amongst displaced persons in Daudu community aspires to contribute to filling".

But this is also reflected in the validation of the findings. What does it mean to be a physical observer, how much more does one experience when psychological participation is guaranteed? This discussion provides new perspectives on the role of the researcher and the questioning of the research process and particularly highlights the scientific meta-level: "The role of research is again highlighted here strongly. The idea is that context must be properly established and culturally sensitive issues isolated through careful research and sifting of offensive material in order to make the mechanism more acceptable and popular with the people. Here, a well-motivated researcher would go into the field clearly with the intention to identify content that can be utilised effectively".

However, the findings generated in the investigation are also extremely valuable. Physically and mentally, the means of cultural performances open up a sphere of social contact, which can provide a basis for positive energies; imagination can facilitate sociability; the distance and proximity of the performing arts can lay the groundwork for openness and tolerance. "In all, the songs, dances and dramatic enactments of the displaced persons in Daudu could be seen as a form of performative reflexivity. In Conquergood's terms, performative reflexivity is a condition in which a socio-cultural group, or its most perceptive members acting representatively, turn, bend or reflect back upon themselves, upon the relations, actions, symbols, meanings, codes, roles, statuses, social structures, ethical and legal rules, and other socio-cultural components which make up their public selves".

In his summary, Shadrach writes that it helps, and even talks about creating a culture of peace. Fine words, but – based on the study – perhaps too fine. However, one believes the facts brought to light through the theatre work; one appreciates the verses of the songs, learns about their dissemination and thus about the reception of the possible – even if, *per se*, this cannot bring permanent solutions. A dose of scepticism is required, but also the realisation that Shadrach is stimulating discussion about an instrument that could certainly have an effect on conflicts. My fears about a healing effect (which he shares to some extent) are that involvement in cultural performances is strongly shaped by women's activities while men are, at best, spectators, material for another discussion about the relationship between patriarchy and matriarchy.

However, his findings on community building are convincing. It is about intergenerational experiences, cultivating diversity and creating lasting structures for interaction in the communities and amongst each other. Shadrach concludes by criticising the fact that this is not taken into account in national cultural policy. "In a precarious situation, it cultural life which includes identities and expressions become threatened and need protection through the instrument of a cultural policy action that is tailored to achieve sustainable development and cultural sustainability".

He argues for pragmatism in cultural policy that is oriented towards the means and possibilities of cultural performances. "The study also established grounds for policy advocacy. Beyond the known fact that Nigeria's cultural policy is an old document which is overdue for review; the study establishes a case of a certain crucial area that must not be left out in the review process. This is in the area of mainstreaming cultural performances in line with the sustainable development thinking".

The study ends with an appeal to civil society and cultural policymakers to ensure that cultural performances are made possible for the management of individual trauma and social change. Shadrach lays the foundations for this and finds

creative solutions to cultivate conflict prevention and peacekeeping through artistic interventions. He uses his analysis of practices in the Daudu Community
to develop a model of collective management that seems to be transferable. He
is familiar with the literature on the subject and knows how to contextualise the
art of performance, gives the phenomenon a theoretical superstructure, and also
uses the exemplary reflections for cultural policy perspectives.

Shadrach not only skilfully dissects literary texts and dramatic productions,
but also grasps the physical and psychological dimensions of theatrical events
and carves out structures from within that in the past have perhaps only been
examined from the outside. His interview guide is clearly structured yet suffi-
ciently flexible to include as much expert information as possible. His specific
research questions have clearly allowed him to acquire a wealth of material.
Shadrach has provided a sound basis for further study.

Professor Dr. Wolfgang Schneider
Founding Director of the Department of
Cultural Policy
University of Hildesheim

UNESCO-Chair in "Cultural Policy for the Arts in Development" (2012–2020),
Member of the Steering Committee of the SDG Graduate School "Performing Sus-
tainability: Cultures and Development in Western Africa"

1 Cultural Performances, Collective Trauma Management and the Farmer/ Herder Conflicts: An Introduction

The history of post-independence Nigeria has been replete with series of conflicts, crisis and violence. From the election crisis of 1964 to the civil war of 1967–1970, Nigeria has continued to witness intermittent acts of violent conflicts. The underlying causes of these series of violent conflicts manifest differently from one geo-political zone to the other. However, the central focus of this thesis is on the recurrence of violent conflicts between Herders and Farmers which has come to dominate the Central part of Nigeria since the return of civil rule in 1999. Benue State is one of the worse hit states in Central Nigeria where the farmer/ herder conflicts keep occurring, leading to the displacement of several communities with other attendant consequences. One of such affected communities is Daudu, one of the communities in Guma Local Government Area of Benue State that houses three camps for internally displaced persons, with others living with friends or relations within the same community. The living conditions of the displaced persons in Daudu accompanied with their memories of the carnage make them suffer trauma collectively. However, in an attempt to cope with the traumatic experiences, they thus resorted to the use of cultural performances as a way of coping and reinventing meaning in their lives.

Cultural performance is an umbrella term encapsulating a wide variety of performance genres evident in a people's daily events and embedded as their way of life. These performances could be those events in which a culture's values are displayed for their perpetuation: rituals such as parades, religious ceremonies, and community festivals as well as conversational storytelling, performances of social and professional roles, and individual performances of race, gender, sexuality, and class. In this way, cultural performances become veritable instruments with which a people move through the world as individuals, construct identity, and build community together.

The fundamental aesthetics of cultural performances serves a bifurcated function; one is reflective, i.e. "showing ourselves to ourselves", while the second is reflexive, which is arousing consciousness of ourselves to see ourselves (Turner 1982). It is in this quintessential role of "showing ourselves to ourselves" and in the aroused consciousness to see ourselves that cultural performances become significant and critical mechanisms for managing collective trauma which is either occasioned by violent conflicts or disasters.

Generally, violent conflict situations or disasters leave behind them a trail of regrettable consequences such as loss of loved ones, loss of livelihoods, bodily injuries leading to permanent disability or scars which are a constant reminder, horrific memories of carnage, some of which irreparably remain with the parties involved. Most times, these consequences include a mass of victims that will suffer traumatic experiences for a long time; either in their individual lives or as a collective within society. Individuals undergoing trauma experiences have symptomatic manifestations that include sadness, anxiety, depression, guilt, anger, grief, fatigue, pain, confusion, fear, despair, loss of self-esteem, and loss of trust. These traumatic experiences necessarily impact on the social dynamics, processes, structures, and functioning of a collective, or collectives. "Collective" here is defined as a family, an identity group or as a society (on a national, sub-national or trans-national level). It is important to note that the excessive stressful experiences of individuals within a shared geographical space become crystallized into a commonly shared feeling of disorientation, hence collective trauma. Cordula and König (2017) outline four collective identity markers which combine to hamper learning and integration process of collective trauma, they include: collective narratives and memories of loss and despair; collective victimhood; collective angst; and exclusive values, norms, and mental models. They argue further that while some of these factors have been discussed in the effort to understand the protracted nature of violent conflicts (see for example Azar 1990; Kelman 1973; Kriesberg et al. 1989; Volkan 1997 and 2004), the lens of collective trauma has not been applied thoroughly enough in conflict transformation.

In considering such an application, it is important that spaces of creativity and aesthetics within a given cultural context are considered. According to Danita Walsh (in Lewis and Doyle 2008), "creativity underpins our health and wellbeing" as an enabling process that helps us "learn about, relate to and evolve with life" and is, therefore, an essential component in keeping us connected to the self and to others. For others, creativity is a means of emancipation, as skilfully executed works speak to the social situation of the makers (Riggs 2010). Citing Angus, Riggs (2010, p. 23) opines that "the space in which creativity takes place can help victims reconnect links disconnected through trauma such as finding a sense of meaning, identity, and place". Angus describes the creative space, where energy, laughter, purposeful activity, the beginnings of trust, creditability, and confidence prevail as "a privileged ground between a community's potential for action and change, and its alienated and deprived members". This is where the quintessence of the relationship between arts and well-being lie. Daudu Community provides the space for creative performances as a place of refuge for displaced persons fleeing from the violence. The community houses a United Nations High Commission on Refugees' (UNHCR) shelter facility provided through a partnership with the Benue State Government and the civil society network in Benue; this provides a sense of security and space for performances.

It is important to note that performances have the potential to tap into our expressive aspects of body, mind, and spirit through the use of music, sound, imagery, role play, dance, and movement. It is noteworthy too that the performative, beyond its entertainment value, portrays a spectacular representation of a culture, and it is a mirror for entire societies, where individuals gain an understanding of themselves in society, and therefore, in life. This means that the performing arts, and of course cultural performances can be viewed as an expression of a culture's emotional state while also providing a conglomerate of forms that are all artistic with emotional outlets, creating a symphony of emotions, a wealth of cultural information from the past, as revealed through dramaturgical enactments. Through the performative, there is created an emotional bond, known as empathy, developed between the performers and the audience. In this way, one can see that the performing arts do not only heal, but also reflect societal sentiments within that healing process. When confronted with social injustice, like the traumatic experiences of the displaced persons, it goes down a little more easily if you have something funny to take your mind off of the pain it brings. Klein elaborates on this concept in the *Healing Power of Humour*: Humour helps us cope with difficulties in several ways. For one, it instantly draws our attention away from our upset. By focusing our energy elsewhere, humour can diffuse our stressful events (Klein 1989, p. 8). It is against this backdrop that this study considers the medium of cultural performances as appropriate for managing collective trauma amongst victims of farmers/herders conflicts in Daudu Community.

There have been perennial disputes between farming communities and herdsmen in Benue communities. From 2011 to date, these attacks became more persistent and consistent with large populations displaced and entire communities sacked and occupied in some instances (Orngu, Ikpanor & Kertyo, 2019). The consistency of these attacks over the past seven years is the longest spate which has also availed a more stable phenomenon to be observed and analysed. According to the Benue State Emergency Management Agency, about 14 out of the 23 Local government areas of Benue State have come under attacks (SEMA, 2018).

Also, in a petition to the Right Honourable Prime Minister of the United Kingdom, Mrs. Theresa May, requesting her to help "stop the systematic killings and displacement of rural farming communities by terror Fulani herdsmen in the Benue Valley of Nigeria, dated January 22, 2018, the Mutual Union of the Tiv in the United Kingdom (MUTUK) chronicled the incidences of attacks in several communities in Benue, attaching gory images of incidences and stating exact dates of occurrence, number of fatalities and those displaced.

It is noteworthy that most of the displaced persons in the wake of the hostilities move to Daudu for respite. Daudu, a community in Guma Local Government of Benue State, has been in the mention of these conflicts not because it is a hotbed for the clashes, but because it provides a threshold and respite place for the fleeing farmers. The United Nations High Commission on Refugees also recognized this and built a shelter facility there to cater for the displaced persons. The community houses victims in the camp and those staying with relations in the area and thus provides a rich variety of study subjects with various degrees of traumatic experiences suitable for the study. It is important to note also that the displaced persons on their own indulge in cultural performances and this forms the basic motivation for this research which is designed as a scientific inquiry into the nature of these performances and how they function in managing collective trauma from the perspective of the displaced persons.

Most significantly, cultural performances are important in managing the collective trauma experiences of victims of violent conflicts as they help victims to attain catharsis, build an intense community spirit, deepen resilience and envision a brighter future.

1.1 Statement, Objectives and Questions of the Study

Individual artists, cultural groups and peacebuilders working in areas of violent conflicts have engaged various art-based methods in conflict management and peacebuilding. These methods include participatory theatre, narra-drama, painting, and drawing, as well as comic books, radio, and television. Artists in every medium – visual arts, theatre, music, dance, literary arts, film, and so on are supporting communities in campaigns of non-violent resistance to abuses of power, and creating opportunities for building bridges across differences, addressing legacies of past violence, and imagining a new future. However, there is a dearth of scientific studies in Africa interrogating the use of art-based approaches in conflict transformation and especially in managing collective trauma arising from these conflicts, particularly in Nigeria. Bisschoff and Van de Peer (2017) posit that the creative representation and aestheticisation of trauma and the reception of such creative works are very complex, in particular when considering representations of African trauma and conflict created outside the continent, through global news networks, popular media, and cultural industries. They contend further that "many representations of African conflict by non-Africans, for example, mainstream Hollywood films using African atrocities as a backdrop, have not been useful in creating a multifaceted view of the continent. Rather they have led to the desensitization of viewers, promoting voyeurism and a type of 'atrocity tourism', both real… and imagined…" (Bisschoff and Van de Peer (2017, p. 5).

Similarly, Chiang (2008) with the work *Research on Music and Healing in Ethnomusicology and Music Therapy* posited that Ethnomusicology has involved extensive work on documenting traditional music and healing traditions; however, ethnomusicologists have neglected to contribute their knowledge and efforts to healthcare-oriented research while Music therapy, on the other hand, has been focusing on the benefit of the patient, but rarely relates its practices to traditional music and healing traditions or non-Western music. Riggs (2010) writing on *The Creative Space: Art and Wellbeing in the Shadow of Trauma, Grief, and Loss* studied Australian creative artists' involvement in working directly with traumatized rape victims. Winkler (2013) worked on "Dance/Movement Therapy in the Treatment of Male and Female Sexual Trauma Survivors" while Harris (2000) worked on "Dance Movement Therapy Approaches to Fostering Resilience and Recovery among African Adolescent Torture Survivors". Other works deal specifically with children who either encountered traumatic experiences due to disability, disease, and substance abuse or have learning difficulties because of disability (Haines 1981; Gang 2009; Kerem 2009; Williams 2010; Coyle 2011; Esala 2013; Breland 2014; Silverman 2016; Olsen 2017).

From the foregoing, it is important that studies dealing with arts and wellbeing on the African continent, especially as they help victims of violent conflicts in managing collective trauma, are carried out; and in the case of this study, cultural performances are seen as a veritable platform to anchor such an inquiry as they also give insight into the cultural makeup of the group under study. More specifically, the farmers/herders conflict is characterized by mass atrocities including brutal killings, rape, displacements, destruction of livelihoods and heritage. However, trauma management services remain in huge deficit in response to the conflict even as there are no medical trauma specialists attending to the psychoanalytical needs of the victims especially in the area under study – Daudu. Despite the several strategies adopted by stakeholders to sustain peace in the region, art-based approaches have received little or no attention. This research seeks to fill this gap by exploring the potentials and impact of cultural performances in managing collective trauma and promoting well-being and peace-building amongst victims of farmers/herders' conflicts in Benue State.

The objectives of this study therefore are to:

i. examine the role of cultural performances in Daudu Community of Benue State;
ii. determine the functionality of cultural performances in managing collective trauma amongst victims of farmers/herders conflict in Daudu Community;
iii. show how cultural performances could be engaged in managing collective trauma amongst victims of farmers/herders conflict;
iv. identify and explore strategies for mitigating the challenges that might come with using cultural performances as a tool for managing collective trauma amongst victims of farmers/herders' conflicts;
v. identify the role of cultural policy and other relevant institutional frameworks in enhancing the effective use of cultural performances for the management of collective trauma and the building of inclusive and sustainable communities.

The study set out to answer the following research questions:

i. What is the role of Cultural Performances in Daudu Community of Benue State?
ii. What is the functionality of cultural performances in the management of collective trauma in victims of farmers/herders' conflicts in Daudu?
iii. How can cultural performances be used in the management of collective trauma in victims of farmers/herders' conflicts?
iv. What are the challenges and in what ways can they be mitigated in utilizing cultural performances to manage collective trauma in victims of farmers/herders' conflicts?
v. How can cultural policy and instruments of other cultural organizations enhance the effective use of cultural performances for management of collective trauma and the building of inclusive and sustainable communities?

This study is significant in many ways. First, it contributes to our understanding of how victims of farmers/herders conflicts deal with their traumatic experiences through cultural performances in time and space. These victims, (that is those directly and indirectly affected), need to negotiate meaning out of their experiences and generate a positive outlook which is needed for their collective well-being and balance in order to lead normal lives. This will consequently lead them to become more disposed towards conflict resolution processes. Government agencies and civil society organizations involved in psycho-social support of victims will also find empirical evidence to support their activities, particularly in adopting cultural performances which are the idioms of the people with which they connect easily. The risk for a resurgence of the conflict on the part of the farmers will be significantly minimized as there will be a less embittered population which otherwise is likely to be searching for triggers to reignite the conflict. Also, government and civil society organizations will find the basis for policy review in the arts to mainstream cultural performances in the building and deepening of national values such as peaceful coexistence, love and unity in order to attain sustainable development. Finally, researchers will find additional knowledge upon which to build or open up new vistas of scholarly engagements.

1.2 The Farmers/Herders Conflicts in Benue

It is pertinent to note that the perennial clashes between farmers and herders are not a problem that is unique to Nigeria alone. Several African countries have experienced these clashes. Search for Common Grounds (2018) reports that violent confrontations between farmers and herders are prevalent and pervasive in Central and West Africa. From Mali to South Sudan, Democratic Republic of Congo to Nigeria, climate variability, environmental degradation, and socio-political upheaval have shifted pastoralist migratory patterns and increased tensions between farmers and herders. These changes have increased confrontations between farmers and herders, leading to violent conflict, deaths, forced displacement and migration, erosion of inter-communal relationships, as well as the destruction of agricultural and livestock outputs. The increased competition for land and water resources further exacerbate everyday conflicts (unrelated to resources) when they occur. For instance, when cattle destroy the crops of a subsistence farmer, it is a direct loss to the farmer's livelihood, and this may exacerbate pre-existing tensions between ethnic groups if the farmer and herder are of different ethnicities, sparking broader conflict and violence. Similar examples play out for herders when cattle are attacked and killed, often in retaliation to destruction of farmland. In Nigeria, the consequences have been severe. In 2008, the Benue State Emergency Management Agency (SEMA) reported that more than 6,000 people have been killed and over 318,512 displaced persons and were living in 8 camps across Benue; 80, 450 of the above number being children. The report stated further that 120 babies were born and 26 inmates died, (SEMA Report, June 2018). This can only mean that the number of people who have been displaced in the Middle Belt states of Benue, Kaduna, Nasarawa, and Plateau put together is staggering. A 2018 review by Forum for Farmers and Herders Relations in Nigeria (FFARN), a group founded and coordinated by the Search for Common Grounds (an international Non-Governmental Organization), indicates that despite the escalating and expanding violence, there have been no systematic consolidations or assessments of what has been done to this point to address farmer/herder conflict in Nigeria.

Nigeria has an estimated population of over 15 million pastoralists (Awuapila 2017) domiciled in the country. Apart from these, several thousands of pastoralists migrate annually into the country from neighbouring countries such as Niger, Mali and Chad. The increase in violent clashes between pastoralists and crop farmers in Nigeria in general, and Benue State in particular, in recent years has been attributed to the influx of foreign pastoralists from Niger, Chad, and Cameroon. The herdsmen often possess sophisticated weapons.

There are a number of factors that encourage nomadism. The Fulani herdsmen often search for a near-ideal condition for raising their herds. While continually moving toward pasturage, water sources, livestock markets, the nature of the terrain that allows for an unimpeded movement, protective mechanisms for their livestock against the vagaries of nature, they sometimes avoid the tsetse flies, harsh weather, tribal enemies, livestock bandits, tax assessors, and hostile social environments.

Apparently, the Benue Basin has a number of advantages that attract the movement of nomadic population into Benue State according to the needs of the herdsmen:

  i. There is abundance of rainfall
 ii. The vegetation cover of the state is made up mostly of grasses and tree shrubs that are palatable to livestock.
iii. There is a network of rivers Benue, Katsina Ala and their tributaries, which provide available water all year round.
 iv. Low population of tsetse fly compared to areas further south of the country.
  v. A burgeoning International Cattle market in the centre of the country.
 vi. Traditional play-mate relationship between the Tiv and the Fulani, in spite of the recent odds.

The causes of conflicts between farmers and herdsmen can be viewed under the perspectives of farming activities and the activities of cattle breeders. Benue State is known as the "Food Basket of the Nation" both in diversity and quantities of produce. Its location in Central Nigeria endows it with ideal climatic and soil conditions for the production of arable crops namely yam, cassava, maize, rice, soybeans and groundnuts; tree crops – citrus and mango. The state is the largest producer of yam, cassava, soybeans, mango and citrus in Nigeria. Over 70% of the population is engaged in arable farming. Few people keep livestock such as pigs, sheep, goats and the *muturu* cattle. The economy of Benue State is driven by agriculture. Families depend on revenue earned from crop production for the sustenance of their livelihood.

Annual farming activities involve clearing of vegetation, which is made up of grasses and tree shrubs that are palatable to livestock. Improved crop varieties are rare and the use of fertilizers is minimal. Consequently, the soil becomes impoverished and fields are abandoned for new ones (shifting cultivation). Similarly, the fallow period, which was five to ten years in the past, is now only two years in some cases. The quest for farmlands leads to communal conflicts between neighbouring farming communities.

No doubt, the massive traditional farming activities in Benue State are bound to have direct consequence on cattle rearing in the State. According to the National Livestock Project Division (2008) there are ten Grazing Reserves in the State, none of which has been gazetted, and which have been encroached upon due to shortage of farmland. Similarly, designated stock routes have disappeared, also for reason of land shortage and encroachment.

Benue State lies along major International Stock Routes that run through the North-East and North Central all through to the South-East, which record very high population of pastoralists during the seasonal north-south annual migration. In the past, these cattle populations merely passed through Benue State. Recently, however; many pastoralists do not proceed beyond the State. They settle in dry season in order to harness the waters of River Benue and its tributaries and the palatable vegetation in the fadama throughout the season (November-March). Consequently, several permanent and semi-permanent Fulani settlements have emerged in many parts of the State. This development is the source of friction between cattle breeders and farmers during the cropping season. Besides, the migrating cattle sometimes trespass on un-harvested crops and rural water sources thereby igniting conflicts between farmers and herdsmen.

The ever increasing population and farming activities in Benue State have aggravated the problem of inadequacy of arable and grazing land. It is, therefore, very clear that grazing land in the State is a limiting factor leading to conflict between sedentary farmers and itinerant nomads. The situation is further aggravated by annual influx of herdsmen and their cattle into the State in search of greener pasture. With the Sahel region experiencing dramatic droughts over the years coupled with worsening desert encroachment, courtesy of the Global Warming, Benue might continue to be at the receiving end of the effects of these natural disasters. More and more cattle crossing the borders into Nigeria from Niger, Chad and Cameroon will end up in Benue State.

1.2.1 Triggers and Enablers to the Conflict in the Benue Valley

There are a number of factors that combine to escalate the conflict among the identified actors. Some of these include: climate change and environmental degradation, depleting arable land for farming, lack of political will to tackle the challenges, and corruption

Climate Change

Climate is a critical factor in the activities of herdsmen and farmers. The changing climatic condition, generally referred to as global warming, is no doubt taking a toll on the survival of herdsmen and farmers business. The desert encroachment from the Sahara towards the Sahel region and other associated climatic conditions have continued to affect the livelihood of herdsmen as they push further south in search of available space, pitching them against farmers and host communities. This global phenomenon is currently affecting many parts of the world with attendant consequences – including the herdsmen-farmer conflict.

Depleting Space for Farming

Constant urbanisation and demographic shifts in the present day world has increased the tendency and likelihood of farmers to move further afield for farming activities. At independence in 1960, the Nigerian population stood at about 35 million people (The Peace and Security Forum 2017). However, 59 years later, it has leaped to about 200 million people and the growth is expected to persist in the near future (www.ncne.gov.ng). Population increase of this magnitude also means a geometric increase in the demand for food products as a basic human need. This also implies an increase in the quest for farming space for farmers. Conversely, industrialisation and urbanisation have continued to claim all available land, leaving little or nothing for farmers' survival. The continued movement of herdsmen southwards in search of pasture for their animals has pitched them against farmers, eventually leading to conflict and destruction. For example, farming along the Benue River accounts for over 20 000 tons of grain annually (Alabi 2015). This same area is also fertile ground for herdsmen to feed their cattle. Thus, farmlands within the river bank areas are the most affected by the movement of the herdsmen – resulting in a number of clashes.

Corruption

Corruption as an enabler of the conflict is a narrative that is popular amongst the displaced populations. On both sides of the conflict, there are actors who are complicit in the corruption that is enabling the conflict. A prominent feature in this narrative is that of money laundering. Corrupt politicians who have amassed illegal wealth find it convenient to launder the money through the cattle rearing business as herds of cattle are purchased and given to nomads to rear at very low costs, making sure that the proceeds from corruption are safe and yielding interest while also legitimizing the accruing profit. This category of persons is found on both the farmers and herders sides. They are said to have used humongous sums from their proceeds of corruption to buy large herds of cattle which they have given to the nomads to tend for them while they pay the nomads a token. Also, in this category includes powerful retired senior military officers who have the links to procure arms and ammunition to give to the nomads so that they can secure their investments. They are also the ones who readily mobilise for legal representations and public presentations since the nomads who roam the bushes with the herds have no formal education. These persons also hire mercenaries to supplement for any combatant weaknesses. It is common knowledge that they nomad does not have the heavy capital needed to finance violence by buying the sophisticated weaponry that is used in these clashes.

Another issue under the corruption enabler is the sharp practices within the ranks of law enforcement agents or traditional rulers who have the mandate to settle disputes arising between farmers and herders before such disputes degenerate into full scale violence. Traditional rulers on the farmer's side, for instance, are said to be collecting monies and other forms of gratification from the pastoralists in order to give them access to grazing lands. However, the land administration system in these areas does not acknowledge that a traditional chief has a right to allocate land since all lands are family or ancestral parcels, except where government has formally appropriated same in due consultations with the people. Such practices set the farmers and herders on collision course. On the side of the security agents, they are said to extort from both the farmers and the pastoralists when it comes to compensation for crops destroyed. They would sometimes collect more than should be from the herder as compensation and then remit only a part to the farmer, both parties go home feeling dissatisfied and this consequently heightens tensions.

Lack of Political Will

The government at all levels has demonstrated near absence of needed political will to proffer lasting solutions to the conflicting claims of different actors in the ongoing conflict between the herdsmen and farmers. Political leaders have failed to invoke appropriate legislations to be backed by action that would define rules and limits for parties involved in the conflict. At the regional level, the Economic Community of West African States (ECOWAS) has a Protocol on Trans-human Movement, though the framework is yet to be fully implemented at national levels. Lack of political will remains a hindering factor among member states. Political will to implement this protocol and other frameworks remains an enabler to the conflict. Kwaja and Ademola-Adelehin (2018) avers that Nigeria's Federal government, in the past, has made efforts to regulate and control pastoral activities, but it appears that adequate political will is needed to enforce laws. For instance, the government is perceived from some quarters, especially by opposition parties, as being sympathetic to the activities of the herdsmen. This perception is likely due to the fact that the President is Fulani, the same ethnic group that dominates the cattle business. Citizens, especially from the most affected states expected the federal government to deal with the herdsmen-farmer conflicts in all parts of the state with the same vigour and determination it showed in similar internal security issues in other parts of the country.

1.2.2 Government's Response to the Farmers/Herders' Conflict

In its bid to manage the perennial clashes between farmers and herders, the Federal Government of Nigeria has tried out a number of measures over the years. These measures include:

1. *Creation of Grazing Reserves in 1965*. In 1965 the northern regional government initiated one of the first attempts to respond to the herdsmen-farmer conflict in the country (Agande 2017). The grazing reserves allocated large portions of land to be exclusively used by herders to rear their livestock. However, the grazing reserve system was not supported adequately. The government was still in the process of initiating legislations to legitimise the grazing reserves before natural factors such as population growth and other related consequences like urbanisation, and migration encroached on these designated areas reducing the herders' chances of accessing the reserves.

2. *Establishment of the National Commission for Nomadic Education (NCNE) in 1989*. The federal government in 1989 established the NCNE and it is supported by the Nigerian legal system. The main goal of the programme was to integrate nomadic pastoralists into national life through mobile basic education and skill acquisition. The programme intended to integrate them into society through education.

3. *The Use of the Armed Forces to Curb Internal Security.* One of the Federal government's immediate measures to address the herdsmen-farmer conflicts is the engagement of the Armed Forces of Nigeria as enshrined in the

Constitution (Land Use Decree No.6, Cap 202). For example, in Plateau State, in 2001, the government deployed a Special Task Force called Operation Safe Haven (STF-OSH) to check insecurity resulting from the herdsmen-farmers clashes. Recently, the mandate of OSH was expanded to replace Operation Harbin Kunama II in Southern Kaduna state whose mandate was similar to that of OSH in Plateau (Kwaja 2013). Presently, many are calling for a total declaration of a state of emergency in Benue and Plateau States as a result of the gruesome killing and displacement of thousands of people in those states. Nigerians also expect the government to activate all the necessary sections of the constitution regarding the use of the military in internal security. This call came as a fall-out of recent action taken by the government to suppress the Indigenous Peoples of Biafra's (IPOB) agitations in the South-East and similar uprisings in other parts of the country. The military was deployed in September 2017 in an operation code-named Operation Python Dance to suppress the IPOB agitation and protests (Fulani 2017).

4. *Introduction of the National Grazing Reserve Bill 2016.* A National Grazing Reserve bill was sponsored in 2016 at the parliament to address the herdsmen-farmer conflicts. The Bill did not survive due to opposition from different stakeholders. Those that opposed the Bill hinged their rejection on the provisions of the Land Use Act of 1978 which vests all powers related to the regulation of ownership, acquisition, administration, and manage-ment of Nigerian land with the state governors (International Crisis Group 2017). Thus, the Land Use Act is an Act of the National Assembly, and by implication, a binding legislation, unless it is amended. State governments and their representatives at the parliament have always opposed any attempt to establish grazing reserves in their domain. They consider it to be usurping the constitutional powers vested in them.

5. *Proposed Cattle Ranching System 2018.* In reaction to increasing conflicts and mass killings resulting from seasonal pastoral movements, the govern-ment in 2018, as a matter of policy approved a 10-year National Livestock Plan at a cost of about 179 billion naira. The plan would culminate in the establishment of 94 ranches in 10 pilot states of the federation. Again, state governments, especially in the South and North Central areas rejected the proposal on the grounds of not having enough space for such projects.

6. *Legislation Prohibiting Open Grazing.* As part of measures to end the per-sistent conflict between herdsmen and farmers in various states, government at state levels began enacting legislations prohibiting open grazing in their States. This, they hope, would reduce the risk of herdsmen destruction of farm lands and the associated conflicts. Benue, Ekiti and Taraba states are

leading this opposition by enacting state laws prohibiting open grazing. On 22 May 2017 Benue State enacted the Open Grazing Prohibition and Ranches Establishment Law (2017) and its implementation began on 1 November 2017. The legislatures of Ekiti, Taraba and Oyo States have also passed Bills prohibiting open grazing in their states. This makes open grazing under any guise, an illegal activity punishable by law.

7. *The Great Green Wall Agency of the Federal Government.* In 2013the Federal government established the Great Green Wall Agency to tackle desertification. This was in response to the 2007 African Union Great Green Wall Initiative that aimed at encouraging member states to plant 8000km of trees along the Southern Sahel to counter the effects of desertification along that area. Continued desert encroachment along the Sahel region as a result of climate change is a major factor responsible for seasonal migration of herdsmen from one region to the other in search of water and vegetation for cattle grazing.

1.2.3 Efforts by Civil Society Organizations

The Civil Society Organizations have not been left out in the fight to find lasting solutions to the violent relations between farmers and herders in the Middle Belt states of Nigeria. International Non-Governmental Organizations alongside their local implementing partners have made inroads in various dimensions. In 2012, Mercy Corps launched a program on Community-Based Conflict Management and Cooperative Use of Resources (CONCUR), in four states of the Middle Belt – Benue, Kaduna, Nasarawa, and Plateau. The intervention focused on working with local actors such as the Pastoralist Resolve (PARE) and the All Farmers Association of Nigeria (AFAN) (Mercy Corps 2017). Similarly, Search for Common Ground launched a program in 2015 to build social and cultural bridges between farmers and herders in Kaduna, Nasarawa, and Plateau States. The program used dialogue and mediation as tools for building and strengthening intercultural understanding between the two groups; as well as supporting efforts towards the conflict prevention, management and resolution as the case may be. Search for Common Ground report (2016) indicates that through the use of mediation, Nigerian-based organizations and agencies such as the Inter-Faith Mediation Centre (IMC), Justice Development and Peace Caritas, Community Action for Popular Participation (CAPP) have been deeply involved in series of intervention with some degree of success that are linked to fostering harmony, rebuilding trust and the cessation of violence in several communities throughout the Middle Belt.

2 Conceptualisations and Theories

This chapter reviews literature and concepts that are related and relevant to the analytical concerns of this study. The literature review here constructively builds on and intends to contribute to a broader understanding of cultural performances as an imperative vehicle that negotiates for collective trauma management, collective healing, performance therapy, cultural sustainability and community building. The chapter also contains an exposition on the theory that underpins the study.

2.1 Conceptual Orientation

2.1.1 Cultural Performance

The concept of performance, as understood by the social anthropologist, Turner, has its etymological root in the French *parfounir* – to "accomplish completely". Turner derives from this understanding the theory that "performance does not necessarily have the structuralist implications of manifesting form, but rather the *processual* sense of "bringing to completeness" or "of accomplishing". In this sense, to perform would be to complete a more or less involved process rather than to do a single deed or act (Turner, 1982). From this perspective therefore, performance would not necessarily mean performing for an outside spectator, but can also mean playing for and with the enclosed cultural collective of performer-spectators or participant-spectators.

From the notion of cultural collective also arose the concept of cultural performance, which John MacAloon defines as "the occasion in which as a culture or society, we reflect upon and define ourselves, dramatize our collective myths and history, present ourselves with alternatives, and eventually change in some ways while remaining the same in other" (in Carlson 2004, p. 23). In another position, Turner sees cultural performance as an aesthetic family which includes such genres as folk-epics, ballads, stage dramas, ballet, modern dance, the novel, poetry readings, art exhibitions, and religious ritual. In all these genres, the media can be both verbal and non-verbal. Each genre and its specific performances are underpinned by social structures and processes of the times in which they appear. Turner proceeds by summarising that the "genres of cultural performances constitute the plural 'self-knowledge' of a group" (cited in Myerhoff 1986, p. 263). In cultural performance, one may "come into the full consciousness of our human capability – and perhaps human desire... all these require *skill, craft, a coherent, consensually validated set of symbols and social arenas for appearing.* It also requires an audience in addition to performers" (Turner and Bruner 1986, p. 42). This implies organized units of events or activity within a society that involves a set of performers and an audience, including theatre and dance but also such social rituals as weddings and religious celebrations. Turner (1988, p. 22) opines that:

> ...if the contrivers of cultural performances, whether these are recognized as "individual authors", or whether they as representatives of a collective tradition, geniuses or elders, "hold the mirror up to nature", they do this with "magic mirrors" which make ugly or beautiful events or relationships which cannot be recognized as such in the continuous flow of quotidian life in which we are embedded.

The mirrors so implied herein themselves are not mechanical, but consist of reflecting consciousness, i.e. the circumstances where those people involved become conscious, through witnessing and often participating in such performances, of the nature, texture, style, and giving meanings of their own lives as members of a socio-cultural community. To Singer, these performances become

> ...elementary constituents of the culture and the ultimate units of observation, each one (having) a definitely limited time span, or at least a beginning and an end, and organized program of activity, set of performers, an audience, and a place and occasion of performance. Whether it was a wedding, a "sacred thread' ceremony, a floating temple festival, a ritual recitation of a sacred text, or a devotional movie, these (were) kinds of things that an outsider could observe and comprehend within a single direct experience. (Turner 1988, p. 23)

In particular terms, Africa's indigenous cultural heritages are a mix of traditional festivities, ceremonial rites, flamboyant masquerades, colourful costumes, exotic dances, and other manifestations that make up the creative endowment of indigenous communities. In the cultural performance family therefore, it is the network of features among the aesthetic genres of ritual and performance that constitute the probing interest of social anthropologists in order to understand the cultural significance and meanings that a performance communicates to the cultural group participating in it – either as performers, spectators or both.

In Africa, indigenous performances are not only cultural but also communal. Amidst the cultural heterogeneity of African societies lies a profuse diversity of performative traditions resulting from the huge spread of peoples and cultural traditions across the continent, and each of these cultures has its rich performance tradition. Thus, a traditional performance, as noted by Nzewi (1978, p. 16):

…is drama, is dance, is music, is mime, is language, and even implicates visual plastic costume arts as consciously organized and exhibited representations. More often it is a combination of any or all of the above in a sequence of public performances which derive its unity from the consistency of its given themes. Traditional theatre, in its social setting, functioned as mass media for every given community. It documented cultural values and trends in oral tradition, and prescribes a cycle of performances. Traditional theatre expressed the socio-cosmological rationalizations of a community and manifested these in stylized modes and observances. Traditional theatre was an important part of the life style and socio-religious systems of the community…

This conception presents cultural performances as a corpus of artistic treasures whose ownership lies with the collective consciousness of the people. The dramatic quotient of the traditional societies is a reflection of their past, present and future – a reflection Ozumba (1997, p. 38) posits to include "…our problems, life expectations, provision of solution based on our patterns of thought and circumstances and stemming from our picture of reality". The reality in most traditional African societies is that the culture and traditions have religious conceptions. Nothing ever happens by chance. Every other thing is directed and set in a motion towards a destination. The absolute implication is that whenever peoples' path meet and an incident occurs, it is regarded as a divine arrangement.

2.1.2 Cultural Sustainability

Cultural sustainability is linked but not equal to issues of social sustainability, such as social justice and equity, social infrastructure, participation and engaged governance, social cohesion, social capital, awareness, needs and work, and issues of the distribution of environmental assets and liabilities. Rather, a broad understanding of culture suggests that cultural sustainability moves beyond social sustainability and that there can be important issues of sustainable development that are missed without a further examination of the role of culture. However, the cultural dimensions of sustainability do not have to be understood as a separate and fourth pillar. Culture can also be seen as the foundation or necessary condition for meeting the aims of sustainable development in the first place or as a perspective through which understandings of social, economic, and environmental sustainability may appear.

Culture has gained much attention in sustainability debate across the world as an aspect of its own and as part of social sustainability. It is often analysed within or as part of social sustainability. Cultural sustainability goes far beyond being social sustainability. Once it is limited to social sustainability, many aspects of sustainable development will be left out if culture is not well included. This is because achieving sustainable development critically depends on human activities and behaviours which are of course culturally embedded. It is of necessary importance to note that culture is at the base for which the realization of the other components of sustainability can be achieved.

Be that as it may, Hawkes (2003:1) sees culture as a fourth pillar of sustainability. He does not only place culture at the same level as economic, social and ecological development, but has given an equal position to the three traditional triads of sustainability. Culture being a pillar on its own, gives it more light in the sustainability discussion. He argues that,

> Cultural vitality is as essential to a healthy and sustainable society as social equity, environmental responsibility and economic viability. In order for public planning to be more effective, its methodology should include an integrated framework of cultural evaluation along similar lines to those being developed for social, environmental and economic impact assessment.

To Hawkes, therefore, culture should be used as an essential element in the structures that facilitate, and underpin effective public planning. This means that peacebuilding initiatives and programmes targeting well-being, particularly of people suffering trauma, necessarily have to be embedded in their cultural contexts and using the bottom-up approach.

Aside the argument of Hawkes as presented above, Throsby (2008:5) argues that, "… the best hope for introducing culture into the development policy agenda is by demonstrating how the cultural industries can contribute to sustainable development, through the contribution that artistic and cultural production, dissemination and participation make to economic empowerment, cultural enrichment and social cohesion in the community". He went further to initiate a set of principles to be used as a checklist against which particular policy measures can be judged in order to ensure their cultural sustainability. These principles are as follows;

i. Intergenerational equity: development must take a long-term view and not be such as to compromise the capacities of future generations to access cultural resources and meet their cultural needs; this requires particular concern for protecting and enhancing a nation's tangible and intangible cultural capital.

ii. Intra-generational equity: development must provide equity in access to cultural production, participation and enjoyment to all members of the community on a fair and non-discriminatory basis; in particular, attention must be paid to the poorest members of society to ensure that development is consistent with the objectives of poverty alleviation.

iii. Importance of diversity: just as sustainable development requires the protection of biodiversity, so also should account be taken of the value of cultural diversity to the processes of economic, social and cultural development.
 iv. Precautionary principle: when facing decisions with irreversible consequences such as the destruction of cultural heritage or the extinction of valued cultural practices, a risk-averse position must be adopted.
  v. Interconnectedness: economic, social, cultural and environmental systems should not be seen in isolation; rather, a holistic approach is required, i.e. one that recognises interconnectedness, particularly between economic and cultural development.

Against the above background, it is critical to recognise that policies tailored around these principles may deliver completely, only to some extent, or not at all; in some cases, only two or three of the criteria may be relevant. In other words, transforming these principles of Culturally Sustainable Development into policy terms will require judgement tailored to specific circumstances.

Considering the above principles, in order to attend culturally sustainable development, particular policies must be put in place for specific situations. From Throsby's viewpoint, the argument canvassed in his paper is that culture can be seen as both a facilitator and a driver of development. The facilitator role derives from the fact that all development takes place in a cultural context, such that the successful implementation of development policies across board depends importantly on the cultural circumstances in which the policies are being applied. The culture-as-driver thrust is based primarily on the potential of the cultural industries to generate growth, incomes and employment in developing economies in a manner consistent with the preservation and enhancement of local cultures. In this thesis, however, it is the "facilitator role" that engages the analytical concerns herein, and this is considered from the viewpoint of "procedural sustainability".

Procedural Sustainability

In order to expand sustainability work beyond a primarily cognitive approach, one useful step is to strategically conceive of sustainability as an emergent property of practices that occur on the ground, in real life. The procedural approach to sustainability focuses on the ways in which sustainability practice and discourse are formed through processes of interaction and engagement. Procedural sustainability is positioned as parallel and complementary to more substantive sustainability that is a more global conception of sustainability that aims to reconcile economic, ecological, and social imperatives (Robinson 2008, 2004;

Robinson and Tansey 2006). In contrast, the procedural approach "emphasizes the inherently local and place-based nature of such concepts as sustainability, and the need for meaning to emerge from within the interplay between theoretical knowledge and local circumstance" (Robinson 2008:75). Procedural sustainability, then, is a strong example of the deliberative, highly interactive and participatory processes Owens (2000) and others support as being a valuable alternative to the information-deficit model that is premised on top-down, expert-driven directives for behaviour change (see for example Blake 1999; Kollmuss and Agyeman 2002; and Shove and Walker 2010).

Research on the design, application, and outcomes of the procedural approach to sustainability has been championed in the work of Robinson and others at the University of British Columbia in recent decades, successfully demonstrating that the principle of sustainability is not usefully thought of as a purely scientific concept, but is in fact inherently normative and ethical (Robinson and Tansey 2006; Carmichael et al. 2004, 2005; Robinson et al. 2006, 2011; Vanwynsberghe, Carmichael, and Khan 2007; Shaw et al. 2009). Theirs is a complex systems approach that stresses the emergent nature of sustainability as a concept, and depends on the beliefs and values of many to collectively shape the sustainable future, and, by the principles of backcasting (Robinson 2003), to work backwards from the desired future collectively described to the present time in order to identify barriers and opportunities and to determine the appropriate path forward. In this formulation, sustainability is an adaptive and always evolving property that emerges from collaborative discourse and practices. While information of various kinds plays a critical role in the determination of desired courses of action, the emergent and normative nature of sustainability requires a culturally and socially mediated process of decision-making (Robinson 2004).

Procedural sustainability is an interdisciplinary approach that "is cautious about strong theoretical knowledge claims and predisposed to epistemological pluralism and the grounding of specific claims in some form of practice" (Robinson 2008, p. 79). This position is highly compatible with social practice theory: "Where conventional accounts stop at individuals' cognitive states and how they change, a practice-based account demands the further step to consider 'doings'" (Hargreaves 2011, p. 89). Social practice theory, which evolves from the work of Giddens (1986) and Bourdieu (Bourdieu and Nice1984; 1977), finds meaning in the everyday routines and actions that emerge from patterns of our social, cultural, and material entanglements (Shove and Pantzar 2005; Shove and Walker 2010; Hargreaves 2011; Warde 2005). Shove argues convincingly that practices and behaviour are fundamentally incompatible units of study: "Whereas social theories of practice emphasise endogenous and emergent dynamics, social theories of behaviour focus on causal factors and external drivers" (Shove 2010, p. 1279). Practices differ from behaviours in that the focus is not on a single actor and the individual's psychological motivations; social practice theory instead seeks "the middle level between agency and structure" (Hargreaves 2011, p. 82) and neatly sidesteps the unmanageable task of enumerating the limitless number of drivers for behaviour that is required by the ABC model which requires an exposition of the Antecedent (the situation that triggers the response), the Belief (our thoughts and interpretations of the situation/event, and the Consequences (the way we feel or behave as a result of a situation/event).

2.1.3 Collective Trauma

This study explores collective rather than individual trauma. It is not concerned with the psychology of trauma, but rather the social meanings that historical events come to have for communities. According to Alexander (2012, p. 4):

> Collective traumas are reflections of neither individual suffering nor of actual events, but symbolic renderings that reconstruct and imagine them. Rather than descriptions of what is, they are arguments about what must have been and what should be. From the perspective of cultural sociology, the contrast between factual and fictional statements is not an Archimedean point. The truth of a cultural script depends not on its empirical accuracy, but on its symbolic power and enactment. Yet, while trauma process is not rational, it is intentional. It is people who make traumatic meanings, in circumstances they have not themselves created and which they do not fully comprehend.

In his book, *Culture, Narrative and Collective Trauma* (2012), Alexander identifies a prevailing lay theory of trauma, which asserts that certain extreme events destroy individual or collective well-being. This lay theory is differentiated into Enlightenment and psychoanalytic strands. The former emphasizes trauma as a rational response to extreme events, the latter articulates the psychological defence mechanisms that are triggered by the event. The psychoanalytic model offers a framework for recovery through the reintegration of the repressed (or dissociated, depending on the specific model) experience. In social practice this leads to an emphasis on truth-telling, whereby traumatic events and their effects are recovered into collective consciousness. A typical example of this would be in countries that had suffered extreme political repression, where the healing process involved some kind of truth commission whereby the denied atrocities of the past were acknowledged, both in their historical veracity and in their traumatic effects on those who endured them.

The South African Truth and Reconciliation Commission is a well-known example of this process. There was a dual emphasis on both revealing the previously denied human rights abuses of the Apartheid regime, and giving a public voice to the suffering of those who had endured these horrors. In this understanding there is a sort of elision of the processes of political and psychodynamic repression. The government did not simply commit abuses, it denied them and sought to erase social representation of these events through censorship and further repression. Survivors of these abuses were at the intersection of both their own psychological defences against these horrors, and the absence of public narratives that acknowledged their suffering. The TRC could thus be understood as re-inscribing the truth of these sufferings into both public discourse and personal consciousness, effecting a healing that was both personal and political.

Alexander finds a common fault in both the Enlightenment and psychoanalytic understandings. He argues that they are both built on a naturalistic understanding of trauma. Although many psychoanalytic thinkers may consider this a misinterpretation, he claims that both approaches accept that the traumatic effects of the event are a necessary consequence of its intrinsic horrific nature. The event itself is a historical given, and the traumatic consequences are an inevitable outcome. Against this position, Alexander argues that historical events do not cause collective trauma directly. The collective traumatic effect of the events on a social group arises rather from the collective meanings that event comes to have. This is not to deny the historical events, but to show how its consequent meaning arises from complex and contested processes of social understanding. Thus it is the meaning of the event, rather than its intrinsic nature, that defines the trauma.

The nature of collective trauma as conceptualized for this study can be seen in Alexander's example of the South African Truth and Reconciliation Commission, where he argues that the narrative of trauma constructed focused on serious abuses of human rights related to the political violence of the Apartheid state. This simultaneously foregrounded physical acts of political violence such as murder and torture, to the exclusion of both the structural forms of suffering (poverty, powerlessness, vulnerability, humiliation) and other form of violence (domestic, criminal). This also assisted in the construction of the ANC as the liberating force and the marginalisation of other elements of civil society that have offered serious attempts to engage and resolve social suffering. These constructions in turn allowed for the initial maintenance of economic equality, the increasing authoritarianism of the ANC government, and now the conditions for the disruption of this narrative in the form of a split in the labour movement and the emergence of self-styled economic radicals such as the Economic Freedom Fighters.

Extrapolating from the South African example above, the interest for this study will not be in the economic and political liberation of a marginalized people, but rather in the underlying argument of what collective trauma exemplifies therein. Within mainstream Western psychology, the notion of trauma is primarily consolidated in the diagnostic category of Post-Traumatic Stress Disorder. Implicit in this notion was the idea of a presumably unproblematic life suddenly disrupted by a psychologically overwhelming event that caused a breakdown of coping mechanisms and produced ongoing psychological dysfunction identified in a specified range of symptoms. This idea has long been contested, both from within South African critical psychology with the alternative idea of Continuous Traumatic Stress and internationally through formulations such as Complex PTSD and Developmental Trauma(PINS 2015, p. 109). All of these challenge the assumption of an isolated traumatic disruption, and explore the possibility of ongoing processes of harm. They allow us to critically engage a range of problems beyond the dominant trauma narratives of criminal violence and sexual assaults, and to consider the structural conditions of social suffering rather than to focus exclusively on the psychology of traumatic events. Thus, while Alexander's book explores the social and political implications of trauma narratives, it critically provides useful additional conceptual tools for critical psychologists in South Africa and social actors in other contexts in which serious social problems such as the conflict studies here intersect with psychological well-being of people.

Cordula and König (2017) outline four collective identity markers which combine to hamper learning and integration process of collective trauma, they include collective narratives and memories of loss and despair; collective victimhood; collective angst; and exclusive values, norms and mental models. While some of these factors have been discussed in the effort to understand the protracted nature of violent conflicts (see for instanceKelman 1973; Kriesberg et al. 1989; Azar 1990; Volkan 1997 and 2004), Cordula and König (2017) argue further that the lens of collective trauma has not been applied thoroughly enough in conflict transformation. This lens shows us that these identity markers inform different stages of protracted violent conflict to varying degrees and, most importantly, continue to characterize the post-settlement conflict phase when the violent conflict is officially over. Therefore, in their analysis, these identity makers overwhelmingly influence the social psychological context for the social and political collective and constitute crucial socio-psychological barriers for transforming war-related identities and successful conflict transformation (see also Bar-Tal et al. 2015).

These four markers mentioned above are further explored in the *Berghof Handbook for Collective Trauma and Resilience* (2017) and is reproduced herein below. A collective narrative and memory of loss and despair is widely shared by many if not all group members. This narrative may be invented or correspond to the real trauma(tisation) of the group members, or some mix of both. The members of this group continuously refer to "the past" and topics of "atonement and guilt" of "the other". At the same time, there is a silencing of shame, guilt and responsibility on the side of one's own identity group: the own narrative becomes highly selective and prejudiced, presenting the own history in an exclusively positive light. An example is the dominant narrative after World War I (in policy and media circles), which portrayed the Treaty of Versailles and reparations that Germany had to pay as a humiliating punishment. Hitler mobilized the masses among other things by appealing to and addressing this collective narrative of loss among many Germans. A Collective victimhood becomes the point of collective reference of a particular group, sustained by "narratives of loss and despair". The narratives of collective victimhood are used to explain and justify the own wrongdoings, acts of revenge in the form of extended violence and the sought-after compensation for the own suffering and loss from the alleged perpetrators. In protracted, violent conflicts, a competition for greater victimhood among collective (ethnic, religious and/or political) groups can often be observed, making it more difficult to de-escalate and transform the conflict. An illustrative example here is the "competition for victimhood" among Jewish Israelis as the survivors of the Shoa and the Palestinians as survivors of the Nakba. On "collective angst", a group finds it difficult to trust other groups and does not believe in a positive vision or a brighter future. Archaic motives are evoked, for example, "…we need to defend ourselves against a tyrannical world". Conspiracy theories are often propagated by greater numbers of identity groups and/or the wider social public. "Collective angst" among the constituencies of the different conflict parties feeds into deep mistrust and the dismissal of positive visions of the future. Illustrative examples are the post 9/11 rhetoric of then US President George W. Bush initiating a "war on terror" along with the presentation of several Muslim countries as the "axis of evil", and the latest travel ban on Muslims (from selected Muslim countries) by the current US President Donald Trump. On the fourth marker is exclusive values, norms and mental models that are characterized by a rigidity of thinking, beliefs in "one" truth, "black-white thinking", "scape-goating", stereotypes, "tunnel vision" and transferences on "the other". Mental models such as "you cannot trust anyone (anymore)", "do only X, as it is normal, but not Y", "we are the people because of past atrocities" dominate social norms, public discourses, media coverage and education. Most of those mental models implicitly give often much needed and longed-for moral or social orientation. At the same time, as these mental models are perceived as "normality", it becomes extremely difficult to question behaviours and ideologies. Conflict parties often use "black-white thinking", "scape-goating" and stereotypes to legitimise their own behaviour and ideologies and to boost their war or violence propaganda. Exclusive mental models often form a breeding ground for conspiracy theories among the wider population, conflict parties and stakeholders, further enhancing "collective angst" and other negative emotions among the general population. Illustrative examples are speeches given by US President Bush post 9/11 and President Trump in 2016–2017, which were full of stereotyping about Muslims (p.4–5). While all four characteristics influence or mutually reinforce each other, not all four features have to be necessarily in place at a given time to speak of a collective trauma. A particular focus should be on the enabling and limiting factors that enhance or hinder resilience and on constructive coping mechanisms on an individual and a collective level.

Analysing the local culture and context-specific coping and resilience mechanisms must provide the basis for tailor-made interventions. It also brings into the fore important cultural differences in expressing and dealing with trauma. As has often been pointed out, for example, in highly collectively-oriented cultures, the very idea of taking the space and room to talk about one's own personal suffering, pain and conflicts within the collective frame of identity might seem bizarre and out of place. At the same time, these cultures may offer greater protection for the individual and his/her trauma specific sufferings and mental health issues. Depending on the role of religion or spirituality, "healing processes are influenced by respective world views, e.g. Buddhism in Cambodia or shamanism in various cultures that favour collective rituals. A collective trauma lens helps to develop a more comprehensive understanding of identity – and roles – formation and allows for identifying particularly vulnerable groups" (Delgado 2019, p. 215). By better grasping the complexity of identity-formation, the field of conflict transformation may offer a richer understanding of human agency and multiple identity trajectories during and after violent conflicts. As the subconscious level of trauma is considered to be as important as the conscious level, both in terms of the actual traumatisation and the trauma healing processes, this research attempts to show the nexus between the conscious and the subconscious factors in transforming violence-related identities. This is where the connection to peacebuilding lies.

There are basically three dimension of peace building (Monsuru 2006). These are:

(a) **The Structural Dimension:** The structural dimension of peace building centres its focus on the social conditions, which promote violent conflict.

It is widely acknowledged that sustainable peace is a product of social, economic, and political opportunities on equal terms, which take care of the needs of the entire people or parties. However, most of the armed conflict situations are hinged on systemic roots. These root causes are somehow complex, which may include skewed land distribution, environmental degradation, and unequal political representation.

(b) **The Relational Dimension:** The second integral part of building peace is to limit the effects of war-related hostility through the repair and transformation of damaged relationships. The relational dimension of peace building focuses mainly on reconciliation, forgiveness, trust building, and future imagining. It strives to play down poorly functioning communication and optimally increase mutual understanding between the parties.

(c) **The Personal Dimension:** The personal dimension of peace building focuses on desired changes at the individual level. If individuals do not enjoy any healing process, it may result in greater political and economic consequences. Peace building efforts must therefore be geared towards treating mental, psychological and spiritual health problems that may follow the end of an armed conflict. Integration, rehabilitation and re-entry measures must be proactive enough to take care of the psychological needs of war victims and the former combatants.

In this study, the personal dimension to peacebuilding bears more to the questions addressed in the research. The basic assumption is that people dealing with trauma will not be disposed to any conflict resolution approach since they are still hurting. It is therefore pertinent that they achieve personal peace within themselves so that they are more open towards resolution efforts.

2.1.4 Community Building

One of the most significant current discussions in performance and applied theatre is concerned with the question of how researchers and practitioners should respond to the concept of community (Kuppers and Robertson 2007, Nicholson 2005a,pp.3–98, Van Erven 2001; Haedicke and Nellhaus 2001). For scholars such as Bauman (2001,p. 3), "'Community' is nowadays another name for paradise lost – but one to which we dearly hope to return, and so we feverishly seek the roads that may bring us there". What appears most critical is the notion of community and the feeling of belonging. In this paper particularly, emphasis is given to the concept of getting together and the potential dynamics of experiencing profound moments of togetherness and solidarity as a motivational force to foster the participants' desire for a better future.

It is important to acknowledge that 'community' is a paradoxical phenom-enon, as it implies a degree of controversy and raises a set of important issues for further consideration. For example, should it be distinguished by its homo-geneous and face-to-face interactions, or by the way people think and feel about their communities? Should it be regarded as an exclusive term (separating 'us' from 'them') or as a conductive term that relates otherwise unrelated individ-uals? Does community exist in pragmatic terms or only as an imaginative entity? As Zontou (2011, p. 77) posits, it should be stated that throughout its history and according to political circumstances the word community has been used with both its concrete and abstract meanings, and as a medium to distinguish but also to unite. To these ends, any attempt to understand community gener-ates the same questions in terms of its ambivalence: community simultaneously separates and unites.

Linked with a number of positive terms such as affiliation, belonging, togeth-erness, connectivity and co-operation among others, the essence of community therefore rests on the experience of unity, solidarity and kinship, but also the feeling of security and stability versus the insecurity and isolation of a rapidly changing society. Hence, the term community has been understood as a system of relationships, ideologies, experiences and symbols which characterize any group of people who are in direct or indirect communication with each other (Kershaw, 2007, 1999, 1992; Cohen 1985). It also describes the feeling of unity amongst people who share the same experiences, activities, characteristics (ex-ample race), beliefs (political, religious) and/or locality, among others. More-over, while authors such as Williams refer to community as a "warmly persuasive word" (Williams 1976,p. 95), and Bauman describes it as "a roof under which we shelter in heavy rain" (Bauman 2001,p. 1), Bruhn (2005,p. 16) claims that "a call for community is often heard in difficult times and situations because it is a pos-itive word which implies togetherness".

Taking into account the above views, one question that needs to be asked is whether community can only be associated with positive meanings. If commu-nity specifically articulates the notion of affiliation and togetherness then does all community belonging feel good? And what is the case for the community of the excluded and disadvantaged, or for those who are themselves included in this community? Therefore, the major problem in understanding community and its lack of ideological integrity lies in the fact that it is connected to a great range of contradictory historical and political meanings and emotions (McConachie 2001; Cohen 1985; Williams 1976). Although, as noted earlier, community is commonly associated with the positive feeling of unity among people who share the same experiences, activities, characteristics (example race), beliefs (political, religious) and/or locality, among others, at the same time it implies a degree of segregation, distinguishing 'us' from 'others'. For instance, as Williams (1976, p. 64) claims in his book *Keywords: A Vocabulary of Culture and Society*, the word community was established in the English language around the 14th century and is associated with the following:

> (i) The commons or common people, as distinguished from those of rank (14th century to 17th century); (ii) a state or organised society, in its later uses relatively small (14th century – onwards); (iii) the people of a distinct (14th century – onwards); (iv) the quality of holding something in common, as in community of interests, community of goods (16th century – onwards); (v) a sense of common identity and characteristics.

It is clear therefore that the term combines a whole range of concrete but also abstract meanings: (ii) and (iii) describe a network of relationships between groups of people who live in a designated area, such as a village. This definition then refers to the geographical boundaries of a location. Additionally, (i), (iv) and (v) indicate the relationships between groups of people who share the same social position, such as class, race and so on, the same identity, characteristics and interests. In this case, community is understood as a notion, the sense of having something in common. On one hand 'community' has been used to distinguish one group from another (such as one village from another), but on the other hand it has been used to combine and connect different groups of people who have something in common (Amit 2002; Haedicke and Nellhaus 2001;Cohen 1985). In many respects, 'community' appears to simultaneously encourage distinction between, but also unity among groups of people.

As Young (1990) argues, communities can operate as powerful means of distinguishing 'us' from 'them' and promote an inside/outside distinction. If the above perspectives are taken together, the notion of 'we' (togetherness) appears to be problematic for two basic reasons: firstly, in the case of communities that have been formed through an act of exclusion, such as *ghettoisation*, or conversely as an act of excluding others, as in gated communities or certain subcultures; and secondly, in the case that an individual experiences 'multiple community belongings', whereby the individual's sense of belonging has been divided between his or her different communities of belonging. In the first case, excluded communities (also known as ghettos) are formulated out of segregation, discrimination and prejudice. Goffman famously claimed that "society establishes the means of categorizing persons" (Goffman 1968, p. 11), and therefore excluded communities can be regarded as an outcome of the 'wider community's' dividing mechanisms. To quote Bauman: "when it comes to designing the forms of human togetherness the waste is human beings. Some human beings do not fit into the designed form nor can be fitted into it" (Bauman 2004, p. 30). What makes the difference in excluded communities is the fact that their members come together as a reaction to stigmatization. Thus, this type of community might not necessarily be characterized by solidarity, unity and allegiance. Owing to its members' similar experiences of rejection, discrimination and marginalization, plus the fact that they are in a sense 'obliged' to accept membership to this type of community, it would be difficult to feel mutual support and affiliation with the rest of its members. In many respects, the individuals are likely to feel that by accepting membership to this community they automatically 'accept' their stigma and exclusion, or alternatively remain without any community: what Bauman refers to as "waste" individuals (Bauman ibid).

However, membership of an excluded community might provoke the creation of another type of community in which members have now come together as a form of resistance and rebellion, and/or as an act of overcoming previous stigma, oppression and rejection. This type of community is also known as a subculture. The individuals who gain membership to this type of community are usually associated with a kind of "collective denial of the social order" (Goffman 1968,p. 171). Hence, the community as a form of resistance might provide its members with ideological justification and rationalization. Yet it can also operate as a defensive mechanism of their social identity and fulfil their impulse for 'normality', belonging and affiliation. Furthermore, it can be argued that the formation of this type of community derives from the individual's response to the 'deviant label' that has been attached to them, and their fundamental need to re-establish their sense of belonging and reconstruct their social identity (Becker 1963). In addition, this form of community is connected with its members' lifestyle and mutual symbolism. Hence, it can be linked to its members' refusal to adapt to social norms and demands. Therefore such communities might attract people who do not necessarily originate from excluded communities but who view this 'deviant behaviour' and lifestyle as a form of resistance to 'fitting in' into social norms. This phenomenon of community as 'resistance' is common among youth or cultural movements, for example the hippie movement of the 1970s (Blackman 2007, 2004; Hall and Jefferson 1993). Therefore this community functions as a means of uniting excluded 'others' who do not approve of or conform to the dominant lifestyle and ideological integrity. The community of people who consume drugs is a well-known example of a community which has been regarded as a form of 'refusal' to compromise with dominant social beliefs.

The other critical issue here is that of sustainable community building. Whereas the discourse on sustainability encapsulates four pillars which are the environmental, the economic, the social and the cultural, the analytical interest of this study is only concerned with the social and cultural dimensions of sustainability. Towards this end, emphasis is on connecting with others, getting involved and building trust. Communities grow stronger when members regularly and persistently do a variety of simple things together that give them chances to connect with others, build trust and get involved in doing things together. The web of trusting relationships that grows from people sharing food, helping others with everyday tasks, and working together to recognize, help, involve and entertain one another makes bigger joint ventures possible and strengthens resilience (www.hks.harvard.edu/saguaro/). People have different interests and gifts so actions that come easily to some might seem alien to others. What matters to the quality of community life is the number of people who regularly connect, build trust, and get involved with one another.

In building a sustainable society, art and culture enable individuals to take part in and help to develop society. In other words, an active cultural life promotes democracy and participation, and generates the preconditions for a good life. Culture brings to society fundamental qualities that are just as important as the ecological, social and economic perspective. These qualities are, e.g. creativity, critical thinking, empathy, trust, mutual respect and a willingness to take risks. What is new is that the very concept of sustainability must include a cultural dimension to ensure that the cultural qualities are understood to be absolutely fundamental to the existence of society and to social progress. Culture is almost synonymous with human action and interaction – and it goes without saying that without it, there is no society.

From the foregoing, the relationship between culture and sustainable community building could be summarized in three broad areas (https://www.un.org/en/ecosoc/docs/pdfs/fina_08-45773.pdf) which include: i) Governance – a well-run set up where local citizens or members are involved in all community decision-making processes with the community as a whole enjoying a sense of civic values, responsibility and pride; ii) Social and Cultural – this underscores that communities members must be active, feel inclusive and safe. It concerns creating a real sense of community spirit where neighbours look out for one and other, are welcome to join in the events and where there is healthy respect for one and other and where all are treated as equals; iii) Equality – the central issue here is being fair to all. People of all ages, races, sex and ability are provided equal access to jobs, services, and education in the community, this all inclusive fairness become a community norm and expectancy, hence culture. It is within this defined scope of sustainable community building that this study is anchored.

2.2 Indigenous African Performances and Cultural Reflectivity

It is safe for the analytical concerns of this study to conceive culture in the same vein as contained in the *Cultural Policy of Nigeria* (1989, p. 5) document which defines it to be "the totality of the way of life evolved by a people in their attempt to meet the challenges of living in their environment, which gives order and meaning to their social, political, economic, and religious norms and modes of organization, thus distinguishing a people from their neighbours". The foregoing underscores the fact that cultural ways, especially as relating to the distinguishing factor of life, are sufficient in establishing the fact that the culture of a people is an expression of the 'self'. This is why even in the Daudu Community studied in this work, the interest is specifically with their cultural performances, particularly the experiences, as they affect their ideals of order and well-being, meaning and progress in their economic, social, political and religious norms as well as modes of cultural organization. Suffice to state that the functionality of cultural performances cannot be overemphasized especially as they go beyond mere celebrations and rites.

The interrelationship between culture and traditional performances basically results to the idea of cultural performances. In particular terms, Africa's indigenous cultural heritages are a mix of traditional festivities, ceremonial rites, flamboyant masquerades, colourful costumes, exotic dances, and other manifestations that make up the creative endowment of indigenous communities. All these have made very significant contributions to the phenomenon of traditional theatre, as they invariably embody the rich cultural and artistic heritage of the African people. This reinforces the fact of the interconnectivity between culture and the creative language of arts, which is the vehicle for the expression of the former. This underscores why there is high premium attached to the quality of art in African region. Instantaneously, one likely to notice that the rich cultural heritage across the continent imbues a robust theatrical tradition all over Africa and this has since put to rest the erstwhile arguments by the Eurocentric scholars about the existence and authenticity of theatre in Africa.

One of the very popular performance cultures common across the continent is the 'festival', which is a quintessential and a quotidian way by which Africans celebrate life and events of social significance. Ukuma (2014) avers that it is common to find a singular festival a potpourri of all the traditional art forms, be they dance, music, mime, drama, costume, masquerades, and a whole lot more. The seasonality of these festivals could be annual, bi-annual, quarterly, or as the case may be according to the historic-communal calendar of the people.

Quite importantly, these festivals are known to exceed a day, and usually run into several days depending on the nature of the celebration and significance; some could last from three days to a week or more.

Festivals in themselves are feast or merry – making events accorded someone or a group or an entire community. According to Amankulor (1985, p. 85), "festivals may be secular like sport or purely religious like the Easter festivals. Both religious and secular elements do come together in festive celebrations and are conceived as periodic observance". Traditional festivals on the continent are avenues for socialization, which engenders a string communal spirit. Also, they are avenues for critical appraisals and reappraisals of a community thereby ensuring conformity to set standards of behaviour and social norms as well as communicating projections for the year ahead. Festivals are significant forms of communal activities that are collectively celebrated by a people within the context of any particular society. Nzewi (1979, p. 96) posits that:

> Festivals in African societies can be in the context of a holiday, often marked by merriment and exuberant cultural fulfilment as a successful celebration featuring elaborate theatrical presentation, honouring a member or marking a collective festive period of a given community, as title taking, marriage ceremony, fertility rites of passage, and forming cycles.

Nzewi's position is congruous with that of Amankulor, both which reflect the assemblage of the entire African cultural heritage that exhibit the act of colourful costuming, masking, drumming, dancing, chanting, and several others in a manner similar to the usage of the dramatic traditions of the African society as the basis of what is traditional African theatre.

It is pertinent to note furthermore, that festivals are diverse ranging from religious (masquerades), occupational (like agricultural, hunting/fishing and farming), and social (like initiation into age grades, marriages and rites of passage, etc.) Nevertheless, it is also possible that a festival could be a combination of all these dimensions. It is also imperative to note that traditional ceremonies other than festivals abound within the indigenous cultures on the continent. These are more frequent occurrences within traditional communities and could range from marriage, circumcision, naming, burial, chieftaincy, or any other kind of celebration that embellishes traditional life. Just like the festivals, these other cultural performances are accompanied by drumming, dances, songs, and elaborate costume, makeup, masks and so on.

Essentially, these traditional theatrics and artistic traditions are the cultural activities and generic preoccupations that are indigenous to the African because they embody and express his cosmological compositions (Ukuma 2014). Thus, the traditional African performance space is replete with a variegated flavour of rich folklore which is expressed in myths, rituals, dance and music, storytelling, puppetry, costume traditions and all the other art forms that abound within traditional communities.

Another prominent indigenous performance on the continent is the masquerade. Masquerade traditions have an age-long history in Africa, and they are acclaimed to be one of the rich cultural heritages in the continent that has stood firm against the onslaught of corrosive modernization. Masquerades are basically for cultural regeneration, rehabilitation and reorganization as they reinforce the union between the world of the living, the dead and the unborn (Mbachaga and Ukuma 2012). It is believed that the dead regenerate for the wellness of the living, and thus, the community forges a cyclical life for itself as it testifies to the continuation of their life force (Ododo 2015).

Masquerades, or the living dead, enact the union between the mortal and the immortal. It is highly ritualistic. In masquerades, the African tries to recapture the cosmic balance between the world of the living and the dead. The masks represent the ancestors who have metamorphosed to the other world or assumed eternity through death. Masquerade traditions are held seasonally, and during the allotted times, various masquerades with peculiar and unique philosophies are believed to visit the land of the living to commune, cleanse, enrich or even to correct their communities.

In African traditional society, masquerades are regarded as the highest and most supreme authority to legislate, execute, enact or evoke all the laws binding the socio – political and religious intercourse of their communities. These circumstances are indeed sacrosanct. Elements of masquerades include the mask, costume, audience participation, music and dance, mime, lighting, etc. The masks of masquerades depict all the community holds dear; from human ancestral masks to plants and even animal masks all in unique contrived forms like fish, birds, elephants, etc. Masquerade performances relieve these experiences and are a great source of African mythico-religious life.

Indeed, the numerous performance traditions found across the African continent are actually an expression of the people's cosmological perception and cultural heritage. This is why Nzewi describes traditional African performances as:

> …the property of the society, its cultural heritage, its functions and exhibitions are necessitated, prescribed and regulated by its society, while its artistic details and organization are been entrusted into a chosen group of talented and acknowledgeable members of the society, according to philosophical establishment of the society in the service of its body politic. (1979, p. 72)

Through constant rehearsal, the community toils and moils, hopes and aspirations, successes and failures are functionally expressed through songs, music and movement. This is because the African artist creates spontaneously using topical issues or situations through the aesthetic techniques of improvisational approach to encode the philosophy of the African people, which is based on their cultural and cosmological given. This is usually done for onward transmission, enculturation and/or acculturation of the society's values, norms and belief systems through aesthetically choreographed dance steps, songs and instrumentation, mime and pantomime, gestures and dramatization, all codified in festive ceremonies. This imperatively underscores the fact that the aesthetic dynamic of African philosophical perception is carefully and creatively encoded in the incantations, songs and music rendered either in solo, duet or choral presentations; more so that "the skilfully choreographed body movement in defined patterns during the performance provides reliable documentation of the society's historical artefacts based on the philosophy that embraces their sociology and anthropology" (Yinka 1978, p. 102).

It is important to note, as Ogunba does, that traditional African festival performance has remained a cultural institution, "a form of art nurtured on the African soil over the centuries and which has developed distinct features and whose techniques are sometimes totally different from the borrowed form now practiced by many of our contemporary dramatists" (1979, p. 19). Clearly, this genre has developed without major restrictions placed upon it by physical limitations or time barriers. For instance, because these performances are staged in the arena style and formulation, without utilizing theatre buildings with all their encumbrances, like demarcations between actors and audience), there is usually an elaborate actor – audience interaction. Furthermore, these performances are done to celebrate life and project the people's worldview and so they are never in a hurry to come to an end. That is, there is no strict timing of performances as is the case in Western contemporary drama. A festival ceremony may take months or even years to organize whilst the actual performances could last for days or weeks. All the artistic endeavours of the people could be brought to bear on the performances without limit. Both visual and performing arts are united in an artistic cauldron in a bid to create a satisfying theatricality. There is no knowledge of and regard for the Aristotelian convention of the unities of time place and action. These performances seek "…to present many aims to be achieved but at the deepest psychological level they are closely related to man's compulsive need and therefore search for sanity and security in a world that threatens annihilation from all directions" (de Graft, 1983, p. 78).

In such an arrangement as explained above, the realistic existence of the universe as an ordered plane becomes central in traditional operations. In this cosmos, God, spirits, ancestors, man and indeed nature are in a continuous consortium, with man at the centre, "forever reflecting and answering fundamental questions bordering on the universe, the relationship between the living and the ancestral, and the position of man in relation to the cosmic order" (Illa 1982, p. 3). In this cosmic balancing, if man positions himself well, his society moves on well; the result is peace, bumper harvest and families teeming with children, joy and happiness. According to Illa, if he is reluctant and stubborn as he is always wont to be, the result is famine, catastrophe, woes and pestilence. Since man's nature is often associated with stubbornness and buffoonery, this form of theatre was evolved to serve the utilitarian function of ensuring metaphysical order and cosmic balance. Illa aptly submits that "…it is no wonder that in most African societies, the functional and utilitarian purpose of (performance) … is a timely arrangement put in place as a natural interventionism, and a mode of religious recourse that will reorder the cosmic imbalance in a universe which man is constantly set adrift" (1982, p. 5). Traditional African performance thus, draws inspiration from the above rationalizations and organizes its presentations and transactional features to enhance its various goals. This position is true of the various traditional art forms which abound in Africa, for instance the Tiv *Kwaghhir* puppet theatre, the Idoma *Alekwu* Festival, the Yoruba *Egnungun*, the Kanuri *Bori* performance, the masquerade traditions and mask dramaturgy of the Igbos, the ever present storytelling traditions across most societies of Africa, the several dances in their various functions, and so on.

The foregoing underscores the vital point that African traditional performances are not mere theatrical glamour but the events dramatized go deep into the very psyche of the people. From the forgoing insights, traditional African performances can indeed be said to have arisen from fundamental human needs which are critically central to the very survival of the African, a veritable blend of the cultural given and its artistic expression.

Against the backdrop of the above therefore, this researcher is of the view that the dynamics of African performances must be experienced on the background of the African context, particularly where these performances are found. This is because these performances are genuinely peculiar just as the people, and therefore the basis of judging, enjoying and appreciating their art should also be same especially as it is a creation from their cosmological experience.

2.3 Performance, Culture and the Building of Sustainable Communities

The performing arts have long been regarded for its potential to foster communities, an assumption that was based on the fact that performativity involves the qualities of collaboration, solidarity and affiliation (Arvanitakis 2008; Kuppers 2007; Nicholson 2005a; Erven 2001; Nellhaus and Haediche 2001; Cohen-Cruz 1998;Kershaw, 1992). In Britain, the late 1960s saw the development of community theatre, which refers to a form of theatre in which community members actively participate in the process of creating a piece of performance meaningful for them. The resulting community plays were based and performed in designated areas in which they provided entertainment, as well as opportunities for residents to participate in the production and shaping of a script (Khan 1980: 64).

Since its early days, there has been an increasing interest in addressing factors by which the utilitarian value of performance within a specific community of locality, interest or identity can have an impact on community building and community empowerment (Coult and Kershaw 1983; Kershaw 1992, 1999). Hence, the emergence of community theatre can be described as a cultural intervention which operated under the principles of "egalitarianism, collectivism and participatory democracy" (Kershaw 1992: 145). It seems that community theatre's intention was to enhance the community's participation and cohesion. It also aimed to facilitate the community's identity reconstruction by promoting solidarity and collective enterprise and by establishing strong relationships and collaborations between the participants and the artists. Therefore the concepts of giving voice, enhancing solidarity and supporting the community to reconstruct a new identity were particularly relevant to the rationale of community theatre (Kershaw 1992: 141–145).

The act of performance involves some form of relationship between the actors and the audience. Together, through a constant exchange of socially agreed upon signs – in the form of words, movement, costumes, and music for the actors, and applause, concentrated silence, or vocal dismay from the audience – each group responds to the other, creating a dialogue as both groups respond consciously and unconsciously to one another.

Furthermore, the idea of community and the sense of belonging (the notion of 'we') indicate a degree of controversy and to some extent perhaps illusion. It is the considered opinion of these researchers that performance is an activity based on collaboration, solidarity and affiliation, and thereby contains the notion of community at its centre. In this sense, social performance ought to be concerned with empowering the community by constantly regenerating its feeling of belonging (see Kuppers 2007; Nicholson 2005a; Cohen-Cruz, 1998; Kershaw, 1992). It is equally important to note that the energy and connectedness that these temporary communities elicit can operate as powerful forces for the generation of a desire and hope for a better future and, perhaps, the desire for a coherent permanent community. Turner (1982: 47) coined the phrase "spontaneous communitas" in an attempt to describe strong moments of people's interaction, as might happen for example in ritual ceremonies or during a football match (Schechner 2002: 70–71; Thompson 2003: 97; Turner 1974, 1982). He proposed that "Communitas (…) representing the desire for a total, unmediated relationship between person and person, a relationship which nevertheless does not submerge one in the other but safeguards their uniqueness in the very act of realizing their commonness" (Turner 1974: 274). For Turner, communitas manifests in profound moments where participants in a ritualistic process connect to an ultimate energy (Turner 1974: 94–130; 1982, 45–60). Turner's communitas appears to be a useful context for conceptualising the moment of "embodying unity" among the participants.

From the foregoing, it is germane to argue that the strength of performance lies in its ability to provide an 'immediate' experience of community, or as Kershaw proposes, "…to strengthen the self-determination of the community, to contribute to the empowerment of community and through that to augment the ideological survival of the community within – or against the dominant socio-political order". One must note that the notion of performance here should be to the extent that it serves as a medium to bring into play the participants' differences and different community belongings (Schinina 2004). Therefore, performance perhaps, should not be regarded for its potential to build the community, but rather for its potential to generate the individuals' desire and hope for community by encouraging them to find their "voice, meaning (substance of their life) and connectedness" (Brent 2004: 222). Performance should thus be regarded as a powerful tool in assisting the individual to realize their desire to search for community.

2.4 Therapeutic Performance and Performance Therapy

The idea of performance having healing properties is not a new issue in scholarly discourse. From the Dionysian festivals where Greek tragedies caught the attention of Aristotle and he had to write the *Poetics*, catharsis was a major effect that dramatists and the spectators hoped for. There are implicit suggestions in the literature surveyed on Creative Arts Therapies that art, music, drama, and dance or movement in therapy can offer a safe place or temporary home that assists in restoration and integration. Furthermore, all of the arts therapies support storytelling, the narration of one's story (or parts thereof), and the expression of that "what needs to be expressed". The creative arts therapies (CATs), including music therapy, art therapy, drama therapy, and dance/movement therapy, provide a symbolic language through their various art forms that seeks to access "unacknowledged feelings and (provides) a means of integrating them creatively into the personality, enabling therapeutic change to take place" (Standing Committee for Arts Therapies Professions, 1989). According to Dokter (1998, p. 16), the creative arts therapies can be utilized to "support the maintaining of a cultural identity, especially in situations where some of that identity is lost or is in conflict with the dominant culture". Refugees may also be able to externalize their symbolized trauma through visual art, music, dance, or drama before they can access these verbally and, upon integrating, experience strength and positivity (Koch 2009). The arts function as a shelter, the active involvement with them functions as taking ownership of constructing that temporary shelter. Aesthetic pleasure can be experienced like a protective cloak, shielding oneself from the aversive environmental conditions, bringing back a feeling of wholeness. Active creation of such aesthetic pleasure can be the means of experiencing resources, self-efficacy and resilience (Koch 2017). These assumed active factors need empirical testing.

Before we communicate verbally, we create sounds, move our bodies through space, and fill paper, walls, or furniture with scribbles and figures. These preverbal forms of communication and expression remain lifelong significant sources of knowledge that embrace imagination, symbolism, and the senses (Chilton, Gerber and Scotti 2015). From the Grecian etymology of the word Aesthetics (aisth ̄etikós) which is "sense perception", one can say that aesthetics examines art, beauty, and taste along with the creation and appreciation of beauty. Thus, from an epistemological viewpoint, aesthetics can be said to be a way of knowing that differs from cognitive, purely rational, and analytic procedures and instead creates a sensory, kinaesthetic, and imaginary understanding (Levy 2015). The German philosopher Heidegger proposed that art is truth (Heidegger 1976). He gave the example of Van Gogh's depiction of a pair of peasant's shoes with the well-worn insides and the leather that implies the dampness and richness of the earth and suggested that this artistic portrayal showed what shoes, in truth, were. Gadamer (2003) went a step further and postulated that art induces an elevated or transcendental state of being. He also affirmed that art and symbols transport us through time, allowing us to travel back in history and bringing past experiences into the here and now, as a holder of memory and history. In other words, images through visual art, music, dance and movement all precede verbal language and can retrieve one's personal past narrative. Thus, the creative arts are in the present, but also build bridges to the past and to other ways of knowing and being.

In Europe and America, creative arts therapies have been distinctly developed into Music Therapy, Dance/Movement Therapy, Drama Therapy and Art Therapy. Professionals are trained and they take in "clients" with who they have therapy sessions over a period of time in order to help them attain the desired state. From literature surveyed and interactions with professionals in Medicine, Psychology and the Performing Arts, this situation is not the same in Africa, or at least Nigeria. Rather, psychologists, from their understanding of the power of music to penetrate the innermost being of a person, attempt to use music cues to facilitate their treatment of a patient, but not that there is a systematically developed procedure that methodically uses music and controls its effect in a way that it achieves "healing" or "recovery" for a patient. As such there are no professionally trained or conventionally practicing Music or Drama or Dance Therapists.

In any case, there is a plethora of healing rituals and rites that are carried out across the diverse cultural compositionality on the continent. This fact lends support to the position taken in this study that cultural performances reserve a potency to enhance trauma management. However, it is safe to posit that both the African and Western contexts recognise the potency of creative arts therapies in negotiating human well-being; the difference only lies in the approaches and methodologies of application or use. It is therefore instructive to examine the various aspects of creative arts therapies that are relevant to the analytical concerns of this study.

Music Therapy

Music has a much greater power to influence collective behaviour through shared emotions and memories. Since the beginning of time music has inspired many emotions, from love, to war and in some cases peace. Palieri (2014) avers that in some rare instances the music itself was able to not only create a feeling of peace, but actually to stop violence. While music is not an end in itself, it is used as a means to an end (Bunt and Stige 2014). In this modality, active and receptive experiences are offered to promote mental and physical health and reach individualized goals. Although our preferences for music are individual, they are grounded in our culture (Bunt and Stige 2014). In community music therapy, a branch of MT that is particularly flexible and can be adapted to different cultures (Ansdell and Palvicevic 2004), therapists are called to be knowledgeable about their clients' musical traditions. As individuals play, sing, and listen to songs from their home cultures, they re-enter a specific emotional state that helps them connect to their inner resources for growth, maintain their cultural and individual personality (Shapiro 2005), and yet be more fully present in the new environment. In this way, they can create a temporary home that feels safe and fosters integration.

The American Music Therapy Association (AMTA) states that,

> Music Therapy is an established healthcare profession that uses music to address physical, emotional, cognitive, and social needs of individuals of all ages. Music therapy improves the quality of life for persons who are well and meets the needs of children and adults with disabilities or illness. Music therapy interventions can be designed to: promote wellness, manage stress, alleviate pain, express feelings, enhance memory, improve communication, and promote physical rehabilitation.

Music therapists work closely with psychologists, psychiatrists, and physicians. Examples of places where music therapists work are in mental health areas, developmentally disabled, general hospitals, rehabilitation programs, geriatric settings, hospices, clinics for people with visual and auditory disabilities, and schools.

Music therapy was introduced in the 1950s and 1960s by Clive Robbins, Juliette Alvin and Paul Nordoff. Music therapy has been a very important tool on helping people with Autism. There are many definitions of Music Therapy. Bruscia (1998, p. 20) clarifies music therapy as follows:

> Music therapy is a systematic process of intervention wherein the therapist helps the client to promote health, using music experiences and the relationships that develop through them as dynamic forces of change.

Bunt (1999, p. 8) describes music therapy as "the use of sounds and music within an evolving relation between client and therapist to support and encourage physical mental, social and emotional wellbeing". Music therapy can help to enhance the quality of life for a person as it allows individuals to communicate with other people in a non-verbal way using music and sounds. Aldridge (1994) describes Music Therapy as a technique which involves the client playing musical instruments or singing with the Music Therapist, Thereby making communication possible. Music therapy makes it possible for a person to communicate.

The music therapist uses instruments to communicate with the individual. They will use instruments that are non-threatening to the client. Music therapy sessions are usually held on a weekly basis and the length of the session is the same every week. Some clients may respond better on a one-to-one basis and some perform better in a group. The therapist uses percussion or tuned instruments, or her own voice, to respond creatively to the sounds produced by the client, and encouraged the client to create his or her own musical language. Instruments will be selected which are non-threatening to the client. The client wants to communicate but is unable to do so due to a lack of expressive language. Therefore music can play a powerful influence in assisting communication. It is used a

> ...non-verbal and pre-verbal language which enables verbal people to access pre-verbal experiences, enables non-verbal people to interact communicatively without words, and enables all to engage on a more emotional, relationship-oriented level than may be accessible through verbal language (Alvin 1991, as cited in Gold et al., 2006).

A pilot study conducted by Grob, Linden and Ostermann (2010) investigated the effects of music therapy in the treatment of children with delayed speech development. The study used an observational checklist where participants with music therapy and no treatment were observed to see if there was a link. Eighteen children took part in this study. They were three and a half to six years old. The results showed that there was a positive effect on the people who were experiencing music therapy. It concluded that music therapy may have an effect on the client's ability to communicate with another individual.

Wigram (1988, p. 44) proposes the following as a useful description of the potential function that music therapy serves for people who have an intellectual disability:

> Seeking to create or develop an alternative means of interaction is one of the primary functions of music therapy. The effect of providing this new means for a person to make contact and be understood has a profound value in satisfying emotional needs, and in building relationships with other staff and particularly with other mentally handicapped people.

Community music therapy is another new approach in the music therapy experience. It is a way of doing and thinking about music therapy where the larger cultural, institutional and social context is taken into consideration. The approach involves an awareness of the system music therapists are working within, it means that music therapy is not only directed towards the individual, but often aimed at changing the system that is sometimes part of the situation of the client. The experience with the study population in Daudu Community can also be explained from this community music perspective in that the displaced persons engage in group *musicking* about their social situation.

Researching the history of music therapy may reveal that this idea is not totally new. In many countries, there has been a tradition either for therapists working within community mental health systems, especially from the nineteen seventies in the United States and many European countries. In Great Britain, there has also been a tradition among musicians to take their art back to the community and give performances as a sort of social service. This has been labelled "community music" (see Ansdell 2002)approach to the use of music in therapy which is sensitive to cultures and contexts speaks more of acts of solidarity and social change. It tells stories of music as building identities, as a means to empower and install agency. A community music therapy talks about how to humanize communities and institutions; it is concerned with health promotion and mutual caring.

Gradually, music therapists have come to realize that ill-health and handicaps have to be seen within a totality, as part of social systems and embedded in material processes. People become ill, sometimes not because of physical processes, but because they become disempowered by ignorance and lack of social understanding. Music therapists have come to see how their tool, music, may be a unique tool to involve other persons, to empower and make visible persons who because of their ill-health and handicap have lost access to symbols and expressive means so important in every culture. Music therapists are now on the way to use music to bridge the gap between individuals and communities, to create a space for common *musicking* and sharing of artistic and human values.

Music therapists are increasingly more often working with whole communities (Ruud 2007). They do not only work with individual problems, but focus on systemic interventions, how music can build networks, provide symbolic means for underprivileged individuals or use music to empower subordinated groups. Ruud posits further that music has again become a social resource, a way to heal and strengthen communities as well as individuals. Musicking thus will be seen as a kind of "immunogen behaviour" (Ruud 2013), that is, a health performing practice, in the same spirit as Pythagoras when he practiced his music at the root in our culture. Whereas this may be true in Western context, the African context is such that music is already a communal art that only retains its aesthetic value when it serves the community, when it resonates with social interests in the society, and these interests are in several ways connected to healing. As Stige (2003, p. 124) also remarks, examining the tradition of music therapy with a focus on musical healing in indigenous cultures will reveal that often, the whole community may be involved in the musical rituals connected with healing (see Gouk 2000).

Dance/Movement Therapy

Dance as a form of expression of the embodied consciousness is at the core of the thinking in this study that attaining well-being from violent social relations and achieving a transformation of conflict has to be negotiated through embodied dialogues. Specifically as it relates to the question of dance as therapy for collective trauma, the expressive outlet dancing creates for letting out emotions and for generating positive energy is considered crucial.

According to Payne (1992), Dance Movement Therapy (DMT) is new, as are all the arts therapies (art therapy, music therapy and drama therapy); however, it has been the last to emerge. It now has, like the other arts therapies, its own validated trainings, supervision of professional practice, and research. At its very simplest, Dance Movement Therapy is the use of creative movement and dance in a therapeutic relationship. Dance movement therapists work on their own or in departments, on hospital wards or as part of multi-disciplinary teams. They work one-to-one or with groups using various approaches and techniques. Conditions differ according to the setting's aims, theoretical views, philosophical beliefs, client groups, staff, and environment. The Standing Committee for Arts Therapies Professions posits that:

> Dance Movement Therapy is the use of expressive movement and dance as a vehicle through which an individual can engage in the process of personal integration and growth. It is founded on the principle that there is a relationship between motion and emotion and that by exploring a more varied vocabulary of movement people experience the possibility of becoming more securely balanced yet increasingly spontaneous and adaptable. Through movement and dance each person's inner world becomes tangible, individuals share much of their personal symbolism and in dancing together relationships become visible. The dance movement therapist creates a holding environment in which such feelings can be safely expressed, acknowledged and communicated.

There are some common misconceptions about DMT which need identifying before going any further. These include the following ideas: that DMT is only for those clients with physical difficulties such as coordination problems; that only people with a natural talent for rhythm or movement should attend DMT; and that only those inexperienced in creative expression need be referred for DMT. There may be clients with all these characteristics in DMT sessions but the referral criteria are not normally on these bases. For example, working with a trained dancer in DMT will require a very different approach from working with someone who has had no dance training at all. The need to abandon technique in favour of spontaneity is sometimes difficult for dancers and can have the effect of de-skilling, when it is no longer possible to hide behind the body's training. Another common misunderstanding is that dance movement therapists are simply teachers who work with patients or clients in hospitals or special schools. They may be qualified teachers also but they are trained in other aspects such as self-awareness and skills concerned with reflection on actions within the therapeutic process, for example, transference and counter-transference issues.

It is important to note that DMT is at times confused with physiotherapy. The fact that both use the body is probably the reason for this. Although DMT does incorporate movement/dance exercises, perhaps in a warm-up, the focus is not on the execution of these as it is in physiotherapy. Both professions emphasize the goal of increasing movement range, albeit for different reasons, and this can be seen as a similarity, but it is the unconscious and symbolic aspects of communication which are the focus in DMT.

Dance/movement therapy (DMT) is based on the premise that body, mind, and spirit are interconnected and that the body reflects unconscious processes (Bloom 2006). Embodiment, a DMT related concept that integrates physical, phenomenological, kinaesthetic, and movement-based perspectives of an individual has been suggested to entail three levels: the embodied self (union of mind and body), the enactive self (living system in environment), and the extended self (embodied self, reaching into cultural environment) (Koch 2011). According to Koch and Fuchs (2011), the body "is the unifying base of the constant first-person perspective that we carry with us" (p. 278). The concept of the self, in turn, is closely linked to home (Meeks 2012). The physical body, too, has been called home, a dwelling for life (Olsen 1998), and an indwelling (Winnicott, 1965). Meeks (2012) suggested that working with the metaphor body as home in the context of DMT could promote individuals' sense of security, control, and comfort, encouraging healthy attachment, authenticity, and an improved body image. Specifically, for homeless and displaced populations as is the case in this study, the exploration of body as a home can assist in creating "a mobile sanctuary in the body, or help them to feel the beneficial qualities of home within" (24 p. 80; 27).

Drama Therapy

Quite often, drama is engaged to promote personal growth and mental health of an individual or group of persons. Drama therapy facilitates the embodied expression of internal conflicts and the rehearsing of alternative choices through role play, improvisation, and storytelling (Haen 2014; Varela, Thompson and Rosch 2017). With roles and masks providing distance, participants can act out tensions in a safe environment, try on different identities and play with metaphors (Rousseau et al 2014). Roles offer an opportunity to engage with oneself from varying distances (example, a human figure is closer to the self than an animal figure; (Orkibi, 2017), which helps clients to create their own save space and regulate the distance as needed. According to Scott-Danter (1998), "the story and issues are recognizable and yet theatre distances them as fiction" (p. 108). This is why Landis (2014) submits that when feelings are physically represented through movement, statues, and sculptures, language can be transcended.

In the 1930s, Dr. Jacob Levy Moreno developed Psychodrama as a form of psychotherapy in which a patient acts out his or her personal issues on stage as a simulation. When watching this group sessions on video, one gets the impression that they are similar to modern-day comedic improvisation, but with the intention of healing. Patients act their way through real-life situations in hopes of either learning how to cope or react differently to problems they are having in everyday life. Moreno was a pioneer in social psychology, but one will not find him studied in a general psychology classes. Through the use of Psychodrama patients are not told what is wrong with them, as would be done in psychoanalysis. Patients come to their own conclusions by voicing and acting out their thoughts, which is essentially rebuilding or rerouting their thought processes.

Psychodrama as a method is very similar to Improvisation. "The cornerstone of Sociometry" as in Improvisational comedy is a "Doctrine of Spontaneity and Creativity" (Moreno 1956). Sociometry to Moreno was the understanding of an individual's place in society. Breaking through anxiety leads to spontaneity that can lead to creativity, a sense of purpose, and healing. In Improvisation, one is encouraged to voice the first thought, second thought, and so on as they come to these thoughts in an imaginary situation. This line of thinking often leads to reversals and transgressions or numerous other hilarious situations aimed at making an audience laugh. Psychodrama, on the other hand, demands a central patient to act out a life problem. The patient works together with a group of auxiliaries to give the patient a very literal outside view of his or her inner problem. The audience can gain from this experience as well through empathy for the real-life characters, from Psychodrama, that are being presented in front of them. The audience can break away from their own fears through empathy, and spontaneity, when viewing another individual's fear. Fearnow (2007) states that people are: Living in a perpetual state of anxiety and anomie, the result of their failures in making meaningful connections with others.

In Psychodrama, Moreno used many dramaturgical or theatre-based terms, each with a function similar to what one would encounter in the theatre. These terms as used in Psychodrama are defined as follows:

a. Protagonist: the one seeking to work out the problem.
b. Director: who is the person facilitating the session.

c. Auxiliary Protagonist: either a person trained in the situation, or other group members.
d. Audience: often up to twenty individuals not acting as the protagonist.
e. Stage: the place set aside for the action to take place. (Blatner 2000)

These terms, but not Moreno's definitions, are universal among theatre groups, hence the 'drama' in Psychodrama. As can be seen by the short descriptions, the practical values of each term are similar to their dramaturgical meanings.

Culture has resided in community psychology in its emphasis on context, ecology, and diversity, however we believe that the field will benefit from a more explicit focus on culture. We suggest a cultural approach that values the community's points of view and an understanding of shared and divergent meanings, goals, and norms within a theory of empowerment (Carl 1976).

Thus, the performative can be viewed as an expression of a culture's emotional state. Performance is a conglomeration of art forms, and they are all artistic, emotional outlets. Psychodrama is a way to empower an individual by giving that individual a point of reference as previously discussed by Bruhn. This can be extended to Theatre, which creates a symphony of emotions, a wealth of cultural information from the past, as revealed through dramaturgy. Theatre creates an emotional bond, known as empathy, developed between the performers and the audience. Dr. J. L. Moreno was ahead of his time. He knew that theatre contributed to a community's health. Before mainstream Psychology understood the assets of theatrical performing as aiding in positive mental health within a community, Moreno was hard at work on perfecting the art of Psychodrama. As the world catches up with Moreno's idea that theatre heals, the theatre's history already reveals societal healing. In genres such as melodrama and ancient Greek theatre, one can see that theatre not only heals, but also reflects societal sentiments within that healing process.

From the critical exploration of the aspects of creative arts therapies above, it is pertinent to sum up here that since these distinctions do not play out well in the African context, but rather a clearly performance tradition abounds within the continent even on scenarios of healing, it is safe to aver that "performance therapy" is an appropriate description of what obtains. Schechner (2002,p. 37) proposes that the seven functions of performance are: (i) to entertain (ii) to make something that is beautiful (iii) to mark or change identity (iv) to make or foster community (v) to heal (vi) to teach, persuade or convince (vii) to deal with the sacred and/or the demonic. Schechner's categorisation of the functionalities of performance is a useful way of conceptualising the performance case study examined in this study as they function to primarily "to mark or change identity", "to heal" and "to teach, persuade or convince". This is directly related to the discussion of how performances by recovering trauma victims can promote social cohesion, positivity and acceptance. Without dismissing the fact that there are many crossovers between each of the above categories, something which in fact Schechner (2002, p. 37) himself acknowledges, it is pertinent to emphasise only the three categories mentioned above are most closely related to the core argument of this study. That is to say, the functionality of performance in this thesis's performance case study lies between the participants'/performers' imperative to 'tell' their stories and by doing so to present their new identities, help their resilience status and send a message to the audience. Thus, the functions of marking or changing identity, healing, and teaching, persuading or convincing all co-exist and interact with each other in the performances with the purpose of raising issues related to the management of collective trauma.

2.5 Collective Trauma and Collective Healing

The term 'collective trauma' refers to the psychological reactions to a traumatic event that affect an entire society; it does not merely reflect an historical fact, the recollection of a terrible event that happened to a group of people. It suggests that the tragedy is represented in the collective memory of the group, and like all forms of memory it comprises not only a reproduction of the events, but also an ongoing reconstruction of the trauma in an attempt to make sense of it.

Collective trauma is a cataclysmic event that shatters the basic fabric of society. Aside from the horrific loss of life, collective trauma is also a crisis of meaning. It involves a matrix of occurrences and experiences that systematically begins with a collective trauma, transforms into a collective memory, and culminates in a system of meaning that allows groups to redefine who they are and where they are going.

For victims, the memory of trauma may be adaptive for group survival, but also elevates existential threat, which prompts a search for meaning, and the construction of a *trans*-generational collective self. For perpetrators, the memory of trauma poses a threat to collective identity that may be addressed by denying history, minimizing culpability for wrongdoing, transforming the memory of the event, closing the door on history, or accepting responsibility. The acknowledgement of responsibility often comes with dis-identification from the group. The dissonance between historical crimes and the need to uphold a positive image of the group may be resolved, however, in another manner; it may prompt the creation of a new group narrative that acknowledges the crime and uses it as a backdrop to accentuate the current positive actions of the group. For both victims and perpetrators, deriving meaning from trauma is an ongoing process that is continuously negotiated within groups and between groups; it is responsible for debates over memory, but also holds the promise of providing a basis for inter-group understanding.

Collective memory of trauma is different from individual memory because collective memory persists beyond the lives of the direct survivors of the events, and is remembered by group members that may be far removed from the trau-matic events in time and space. These subsequent generations of trauma survi-vors, that never witnessed the actual events, may remember the events differently than the direct survivors, and then the construction of these past events may take different shape and form from generation to generation. Such collective memory of a calamity suffered in the past by a group's ancestors may give rise to a "chosen trauma" dynamic that weaves the connection between trauma, memory and on-tological security (Volkan, 1997). These chosen traumas are conceptualized as narratives emphasizing that 'walking through blood' is necessary on the path to freedom, independence and group security (Resendeand Budryte 2014). The creation and maintenance of meaning comprises a sense of self-continuity, a connection between the self, others and the environment (Baumeister and Vohs 2002; Heine et al., 2006), and the feeling that one's existence matters. It is a pro-cess of identity construction that comprises the sense of self-esteem, continuity, distinctiveness, belonging, efficacy, and ultimately a sense of meaning (Vignoles et al., 2006). Accordingly, the current article relies on these principles to trace the process of meaning-making following historical trauma at the collective level and among both victim and perpetrator groups.

For victims of collective trauma, Hirschberger (2018) argues, meaning is es-tablished by: (a) passing down culturally-derived teachings and traditions about threat that promote group preservation; (b) these traditions of threat amplify existential concerns and increase the motivation to embed the trauma into a symbolic system of meaning; (c) trauma fosters the sense of a collective self that is trans-generational thereby promoting a sense of meaning and mitigating ex-istential threat; (d) the sense of an historic collective self also increases group cohesion and group identification that function to create meaning and alleviate existential concerns; (e) the profound sense of meaning that is borne out of col-lective trauma perpetuates the memory of the trauma and the reluctance to close the door on the past; (f) Over time collective trauma becomes the epicentre of group identity, and the lens through which group members understand their social environment.

For members of perpetrator groups, collective trauma represents an 'identity threat' (Branscombe et al., 1999), as it creates tension between the desire to view the group in a positive light (Tajfel and Turner 1979), and the acknowledgement of severe moral transgressions in its past. The inability to reconcile the character of the group in the present with its character in the past may motivate group members, primarily high identifiers, to perceive an historical discontinuity of the group that serves to distance present group members from past offenders (Roth et al., 2017). Sometimes this discontinuity is reflected in the motivation to close the door on history and never look back (Imhoff et al., 2017), and sometimes the thorny chapters of a group's history are glossed over creating an uncomfortable gap in collective memory – an absence suggesting a presence. Members of perpetrator groups may deal with the dark chapter in their history by thoroughly denying the events, disowning them and refusing to take any responsibility for them. But, more often than not, reactions to an uncomfortable history will take on a more nuanced form with group members reconstructing the trauma in a manner that is more palatable, and representing the trauma in a manner that reduces collective responsibility. In some cases, the dissonance between current group values and past behaviour are so great that disaffiliation from the group remains the only viable option (Čehajić and Brown 2010; Hirschberger et al., 2016b).

Understanding the impact of trauma on collective meaning becomes even more complex when considering what Primo Levi defined as the 'gray zone' (Levi 1959) – a nebulous area wherein the distinction between victims and perpetrators is not always clear cut, and victims may behave as perpetrators and perpetrators are victims. Members of groups that exist in this region of collective memory are often motivated to defensively represent their history in a manner that highlights their sacrifice and downplays their crimes (Bilewicz et al, 2014; Hirschberger et al, 2016b). These groups may also engage in competitive victimhood dynamics with other groups demanding to be recognized as the veritable victim (Noor et al 2012).

The need to come to terms with a dark past represents a crisis of meaning that must be resolved for the group to deconstruct and reconstruct its sense of collective self and assume an identity that offers continuity, coherence and significance is quite paramount. The memory of historical crimes threatens fundamental values, current notions of self-worth, and the sense of having a constructive collective purpose (Baumeister 1991; Vignoles et al., 2006). The quest for meaning must, therefore, involve the reconstruction of these basic elements.

This analysis of meaning borne out of trauma for both victim and perpetrator groups offers the provocative suggestion that trauma is not merely a destructive event, but also an irreplaceable ingredient in the construction of collective meaning. Accordingly, for victim groups there may be secondary gains to collective trauma, that are often overlooked, that function to keep the memory of trauma alive, and lead subsequent generations to incorporate the trauma into their collective self. For perpetrator groups, the trauma functions as a catalyst that stimulates the construction of a new social representation that, if successful, can support a collective self that acknowledges past transgressions in a manner that is neither defensive nor crippling; one that promotes positive social identity (example, Vignoles et al., 2006) predicated on the triumph over past failings.

2.6 Nigeria's Cultural Policy, the Arts and Culture in Social Transformation

The National Cultural Policy of Nigeria, which came in being through a military decree in 1988, is generally regarded as an instrument for the promotion of national identity and the unity of the country despite her multifarious ethnic nationalities, as well as of communication. Also, the provisions made by government permit the various expressions of cultural values, and heritage widely recognised as the most important factor in defining the national and ethnic cultures in Nigeria.

The policy document is divided into three broad parts with each part having its own sub-headings. Part I consists of the cultural policy and methods of implementation. Part II entitled "Focus of implementation" targets specifically the areas of Education, The Arts, Tourism and Mobility of People, Mass Media and General Focus. Part III which is the last, entitled Administration and Finance, addresses the administration and financing of culture.

The objectives of the policy document are itemised as follows:

i. The policy shall serve to mobilise and motivate the people by disseminating and propagating ideas which promote national pride, solidarity and consciousness.

ii. The policy shall serve to evolve from our plurality, a national culture, the stamp of which will be reflected in African and world affairs.

iii. The policy shall promote an educational system that motivates and stimulates creativity and draws largely on our tradition and values, namely: respect for humanity and human dignity, for legitimate authority and the dignity of labour, and respect for positive Nigerian moral and religious values.

iv. The policy shall promote creativity in the fields of arts, science and technology; ensure the continuity of traditional skills and sports and their progressive updating to serve modern development needs as our contribution to world growth of culture and ideas.

v. The policy shall establish a code of behaviour compatible with our tradition of humanism and a disciplined moral society.

vi. The policy shall sustain environmental and social conditions which enhance the quality of life, produce responsible citizenship and an ordered society.

vii. The policy shall seek to enhance the efficient management of national resources through the transformation of the indigenous technology, design-resources and skills.

viii. The policy shall enhance national self-reliance and self-sufficiency, and reflect our cultural heritage and national aspiration in the process of industrialisation.

The fourth section of the document outlines the methods of policy implementation in a four point approach comprising of:

i. Preservation of culture
ii. Promotion of culture
iii. Presentation of culture and
iv. The establishment of administrative structure and the provision of funds for its implementation

However, considering the relatively long period of its birth (1988) and the way in which it came into existence (military decree), the document has been a subject of critical analyses which point our inadequacies of content, its obsolete nature and the lack of current with recent developments in the discourse and management of culture. To Anyanwu (2019) for instance, "it must be pointed out however that the Cultural Policy falls short in the area of its failure to consider how to relate with the outside world, especially Nigerians/Africans in Diaspora". Further, Akerele (2011) observes that "action needs to be taken to enhance culture as opposed to a list of theoretical orientations contained in the National Policy on Culture". In this case, the quintessential relationship between culture and national development is brought to bear.

The needs for a well-established deliberate documentation on cultural heritage, as well as a need for a well organised and carefully executed plan for heritage restoration and preservation stand out amongst what could be considered as immediate lines of action. This will set the precedential benchmark for all cultural production and consumption, particularly amongst young people and also mitigate the effect of modernization on those who are susceptible to foreign culture assimilation at the expense of theirs.

There are inherent challenges with the National Cultural Policy of Nigeria in respect to processes of social transformation, which denotes a fundamental change in society. Transformation connotes an experience of progress – the continuous unfolding of improvement in society. This has to be located in the understanding of where society was and where it is now and the likely possibility of its transition to another level in its elements.

It is to be expected that Nigeria being signatory to various cultural conventions including, those conventions will be brought to be on the cultural sector; as it is that is only to be desired. International conventions that Nigeria is signatory to include:

1. Convention Concerning the Protection of the World Cultural and Natural Heritage, Paris 1972.
2. The 1970 UNESCO Convention on the Means of Prohibiting and Preventing the Illicit Import, Export and transfer of ownership of Cultural Property
3. The Berne Convention on the Protection of Literacy and Artistic Works
4. The Rome Convention on the Protection of Performers, Phonogram Producers and Broadcasting Organizations
5. Second Protocol to the Convention for the Protection of Cultural Property in the Event of Armed Conflict
6. UNIDROTT Convention of Stolen or Illegally Exported Cultural Objects, Rome, 1995
7. The UNESCO Convention on the Protection of the Underwater Cultural Heritage, Paris, 2001
8. Convention for the Safeguarding of the Intangible Cultural Heritage, Paris, 2003
9. The 2005 Convention for the Protection and Promotion of the Diversity of Cultural Expressions ratified by Nigeria in 2008.

However, the problem with these conventions is that Nigeria is yet to domesticate most of them in line with section 12 of the Constitution and there is insufficient legal framework, financing and infrastructure to implement the conventions. Most fundamentally, our archaic cultural policy does not embrace many of the conventions. For example, the 2005 Convention for the Protection and Promotion of the Diversity of Cultural Expressions, demands regular review of cultural policies but since 2008 when Nigeria ratified the convention, there has been no clear review of our cultural policy.

Specifically to challenges of preservation, protection and promotion of Nigeria's cultural heritage, Asia (2019) highlights them to include:

1. Obsolete policy document
2. Inadequate funding and budgetary allocation
3. Failure of government to implement the policy on town planning and development of estates
4. Merger of ministry of information with culture which has politicized the ministry
5. Security challenges and conflicts.
6. Appointment of people to head cultural ministries without consultation with cultural administrators
7. Lack of adequate data on cultural expression
8. Globalization and civilization
9. Religion-cultural objects are burnt and despised in the name of religion
10. Our penchant for foreign cultures

This indicates that the cultural sector in Nigeria, both at the state and societal level is not primed for social transformation.

In considering the question of what impact cultural policy can have on changes to government structure vis-à-vis the role of art and artists in the transformation of society, Schneider and Gad (2014, p. 5) posit that:

> "it is not primarily about money, but social relevance; it is not about representation, but intervention. It is no longer just about local art education, regional support structures or national programmes for arts education. Now it is also about …culture as a development factor…" They contend further that culture is viewed as a source for the development of society. Accordingly, the task of cultural policy is to create and support structures that mobilise people's creativity and thus ensure well-being, innovation and pluralism. Cultural policy needs goals that could provide a basis for a successful life. Implementation of these goals requires strategies to be set for state and society (Schneider and Gad, 2014, p. 6)

2.7 Theories

Broadly, two theories anchor this work and they include cultural performance theory and social practice theory. They are considered relevant in that the cultural performance theory anchors the analysis and discussion of the cultural performances of the displaced persons and the well-being function these performances play amongst them, whereas the social practice theory is addressed to the concerns with the quintessence of cultural performance in advancing conflict transformation and cultural sustainability discourse and praxis. The two theories are elaborately explored here below.

2.7.1 Cultural Performance Theory

Discourses around cultural performance theory provide insights into appreciating culture within daily endeavours and interactivity of man in his environment. Theorizing cultural performance indeed helps to conceptualize culture as the centre of hegemonic, or dominating, messages and revealing the hierarchical structure of society through lived experience. This places culture as the current running through all of human activity in the various spheres of life.

The relationship of culture and performance is therefore that of a coexisting entity, mutually complimenting each other, and not a means to an end. It is instructive to note the words of Ficher-Lichte (2004) who avers that:

> We rather have to come to understand that culture is also, if not in the first place, performance. It can hardly be overlooked to what an extent culture is brought forth as an in performance – not only in the performances of the different arts but also, and foremost in performances of rituals, festivals, political rallies, sport competitions, games, fashion shows and the like – performances which, in a mediatized form, reach out to a million of people.

In the above excerpt lies the quintessence of performance as bedrock for the study of human communication. Littlejohn, Stephen W and Karen A. Floss (2009) opine that performance theory views humans as *Homo-narrans*, or creatures who communicate through stories as a way of crafting their social world and making meaning of it. Performance therefore implies an act of doing, practice, and theatricality, while simultaneously encompassing both the subject of research and the method of doing research.

Created from perspectives on human behaviour, culture, and ritual, cultural performance theory explores the relationship between the foundations of human experience: community, culture, and performance. It also serves as a challenge to traditional theory by bringing together differing domains of knowledge – the objective, scientific, and observable – with the embodied, practical, and everyday. Cultural performance theory radicalizes, or identifies as the root issue, the binary opposition between theory and practice by providing a model of communicative practice in which culture and performance are inextricably joined and integral to the communal experience of everyday life.

The term cultural performance refers to discrete events, or cultural performances that can be observed and understood in any cultural structure. These events include, for example, traditional theatre and dance, concerts, recitations, religious festivals, weddings, and funerals, all of which possess certain characteristics: limited time span, a beginning and an end, a set of performers, an audience, a place and occasion, and an organized program of activity. Again,

Fischer-Lichte (2004) avers that performances are characterized by their *eventness*. The specific mode of experience they allow for is a particular form of liminal experience. For the analytical concerns of this study, the question of liminality in performances is further explored below alongside "reflexivity" on the part of the performers and those who ethnographically explore them.

Liminality

Liminality accounts for the in-between phase of transitioning from one reality to another. It is believed that so much happens within this phase that impacts immensely in shaping the new reality to emerge. Arnold van Gennep first conceptualised this idea in his seminal work, *Rités de Passàge* (1909) (translated to English in 1969) where the notion of liminality is hinged on the twin idea of "encompassing marginal space" and "threshold crossing" (Jain 2005). Gennep (1969) posited that:

> ..."crossing the threshold" means incorporating oneself into a new world. Therefore, it is an important act in weddings, adoption, ordination, and funerary ceremonies... One will note that rites carried out on the threshold itself are marginal rites. As rites of separation from the previous world, there are rites of "purification" (one washes, one cleans oneself, etc.), then rites of aggregation (presentation of salt, sharing a meal, etc.). The threshold rites are thus not strictly speaking "alliance" rites, but rites to prepare for alliance, preceded themselves by rites to prepare for the marginal space. (Turner 1977)

The idea in the above excerpt can simply be summed up as an embedded interest in margins, borders and transitions.

By the performative turn, it was Victor Turner, a British anthropologist, who popularised the threshold crossing idea of Gennep to explain the transitioning experienced in the rituals of "small-scale pre-industrial" societies; rituals carried out to signify a transition from one social identity to another – from child to adult, single to married, citizen to king, living to dead. It is against this background that liminality is consider to be (Skjoldager-nielsen & Edelman 2014) "a transitory and precarious phase between stable states, which are marked off by conceptual, spatial and/or temporal barriers, within which individuals, groups and/or objects are set apart from society and/or the everyday". In reference to individuals or their groups, therefore, people in luminal state lose their former symbolic status, but they are yet to attain a new significance. This means that they exist in a state of flux, "an in-between of potent but dangerous formlessness". Liminality, thus, denotes an undefined spatio-temporal spectrum within which transformation, change, modification or evolution is experience and achieved.

From the rituals both Van Gennep and Turner studied over time, they noticed three stages in their unfolding patterns. Van Gennep referred to these stages as "rites of separation", "rites of transition", and "rites of incorporation" while Turner described them as "pre-liminal, liminal, and post-liminal".

In the first stage which is "rites of separation" or "pre-liminal", participants (that is the candidates for initiation) experience a stripping of their stable or established social identity from them just as they were frequently (or over a defined period of time) set apart and secluded from the rest of the community. Symbolically, this meant that by losing their known social identity, the candidates for initiation became dead to the society. The second stage, "rites of transition" or "luminal", took place during the period of being isolated from the society. At this time, two things were central: first, a systematic conditioning that required strict adherence to a strenuous (and in some cases excruciating) sequence of activities (which could be tests), religiously enforced by a master-in-charge; and second, "a sense of impersonal, unstructured, but hugely potent commonality amongst the group of initiands that Turner called 'communitas'" (Skjoldager-nielsen & Edelman 2014).

The third and final phase, "rites of incorporation" or "post-liminal", was a symbolic rebirth. The candidates for initiation earlier considered dead to the society through separation, having undergone transition are now reintroduced into the society with their freshly forged identities and the process of reintegration begins as they assume their new roles with new perspectives to events and order in the society.

In addition to the personal transitions these rites engender amongst the participants, Turner saw the process fitting to what he describes as "social dramas", which refers to the ways in which societies could use rituals to creatively respond to crises such as death of kings, schisms, or other disasters. Thus, liminality resides in this middle, in-between undefined space that is lacking in structure, thereby making the emergence of new social realities possible.

In order to connect with modernity, this phenomenon of liminality established on the basis of the practices of pre-industrial societies, Turner sought a new path through his collaboration with a New York theatre director and theorist, Richard Schechner. The central question to Turner was what happened to the liminal in modern societies where social structures were not so clearly defined in a way that they could be discarded and remade, even in ritual; what was obvious to him was that social creativity was still very much in need in modern commercial society, yet he could not observe the three-part structure of experience (Skjoldager-nielsen & Edelman, 2014).

However, recent scholarship has made attempts at exploring ways in which the effect of witnessing a performance can serve for both social and individual change, as well as forms that combine the two (Skjoldager-nielsen & Edelman 2014). Some of these works are explored here below.

The first work of interest here is the Transformative Power of Performance (Fischer-Lichte 2008), where it is argued that there is a particular potency to the presence ofthe actor and audience together in the performance space; "the radical concept of presence" (p. 99). Fischer-Lichte understands performance as an event that generates itself through the bodily co-presence and energetic exchanges (feedback) of its participants (actors and spectators alike); the ephemeral and transient factors making the performance event inherently unpredictable and unrepeatable. Through the performance event, the clearly defined entities which are easily identified with symbolic statuses such as spectator and actor, arts and life, ritual and theatre, can be destabilised. It is, thus, these contingencies of performances which "enable experiences that always carry a liminal dimension" (p.176).

Fischer-Lichte argues further that liminal experience first emerges in the body as a change to the physiological, energetic, affective and motoric state (p.177). This level of the spectator's experience is connected to the above mentioned radical presence of the actor, which evokes in the spectators a similar notion of presence "as embodied mind in a constant process of becoming (p.99), followed by a profound sense of joy and fulfilment. Although Fischer-Lichte understands this radical presence as a transient, intense and extraordinary experience that rejects dichotomies, it is not included in her examples of the liminal. Rather, what can be deduced from her examples is that the liminal tends to be less associated with the joyful. Her examples are rather experimental performances that disregard conventional behaviour by, for instance, inviting the audience to partake in a communal abolishment of social norms or letting them bear witness to a performer's suffering or self-injury. In these liminal moments, "established standards (of behaviour) are no longer valid and new ones are yet to be formulated (p.176). This means then that liminal experience is often coupled with transgressions of individual and social limits and as such retain the quality of unpleasantness and peril associated with the Tunerian sense of liminality.

There is a critical issue stemming out from the foregoing, and that is the understanding of the actor-spectator relationship; perhaps, a second issue will be the question, "whose liminality?", if the Gennep and Turner three-stage pattern is still to anchor the understanding of the liminality discourse. Performance in the African context is rather more participatory and thus blurs the lines in the actor-spectator binaries as is the case in Western style performance. This fact is not lost on Western scholars, so to discourse performance from an exclusively Western viewpoint as Fischer-Lichte does above does not help in decolonising the discourse.

Another work of interest in theorising liminality is *Utopia in Performance*(Dolan 2005). In this book, Dolan argues that "the political potential of performance comes not in its ability to put forward concrete proposals, but rather through the glimpse it offers of a sense of social connectedness that she equates with the Tunerian communitas" (Skjoldager-nielsen & Edelman 2014). Therefore, the core issue for her is that performance offers "moments of liminal clarity and communion, fleeting, briefly transcendent bits of profound human connections" (Dolan 2005, p. 168).

Reflexivity

Reflexivity is the process of reflection, which takes itself as the object; in the most basic sense, it refers to reflecting on *oneself* as the *object* of provocative, unrelenting thought and contemplation. Reflexivity makes a claim to self-reference (Charlotte 1998). According to Myerhoff and Ruby (1982), reflexivity generates "heightened awareness and vertigo, the creative intensity of a possibility that loosens us from habit and custom and turns back to contemplate ourselves". Reflexivity is a technical term that permeates critical literary discourse and social science research, as well as aspects of the autobiographical life of regular people. Reflexivity is an aspect of social and anthropological writing and research; however, its interest for literary studies lies in its universal application. Anthropological works depend on their meticulous note taking, and their success is determined by their rhetorical competence which occurs in monographs and self-exposing diaries, travel journals, and so on.

From the point of view of the author, narrator, or anthropologist-writer, reflexivity refers to what is otherwise known as the author's or discipline's *self-consciousness*. The word *reflexive* comes from the Latin *reflexus*, meaning "bent back", which in turn comes from *reflectere*– to reflect. Reflexivity is a process which has imbued post-structural anthropological discourse with a focus on the narrator's proverbial *self*: self-examination, self-strategies, self-discovery, self-intuition, self-critique, self-determination, selfhood. The semantic content of *self* is not clear; however, there is a consensus that it makes a general reference to the debate over objectivity and subjectivity (Turner 1988). Responses to the attempts apparently raised by reflexivity involve attempts to ensure objectivity through reducing or controlling the effects of the researcher on the research situation. Such attempts include maintaining distance through using observation and other methods in which interaction is kept to a minimum or is highly controlled (Davies 1998). These approaches have been identified with positivist and naturalist methodologies, respectively (Hammerseley and Atkinson 1983). It therefore holds that the most rigid, objectivist approaches are often accompanied by a great deal of reflexivity.

In modern anthropological discourse, reflexivity is very much associated with the kind of experimental works that have come out of current anthropology: especially the rise of diary writing and the emergence of auto-ethnographies, in which the self is explored through a focal subjective lens in light of one's social history. Reflexivity in anthropology refers to how the studied 'object' of research reacts towards fieldwork, to mould new epistemological areas of research. In modern anthropology, studied objects are seen through the hall of mirrors of dialogue and self-reflection, and granted a (post-colonial and post-modern) *voice* within the text. It is no longer the question of being confronted with the text written by an anthropologist, as much as the discourse of a native person who dares to speak his or her own story within the story of the anthropologist. There have been cases of native people bringing lawsuits against anthropologists, for misusing and misinterpreting their information in the field (Dwyer 1999). In other words, reflexivity refers to how personal an anthropological text really becomes. Personal history is not the only element which influences objectivity. The social interaction between the ethnographer and his subjects of study influences the way in which an ethnographic account is constructed.

Participant observation is characterised by a 'stepping in and out of the context', a sort of distance between self, vis-à-vis the subject of study. On one hand, one has to get 'native' and get into the mood of the research through participation. On the other hand, one needs to distance oneself to ponder and examine, through observation (Powdermaker 1966). It is critical that research be based on pragmatic and realist ontology; however, the personal element cannot be removed from the equation.

Within the parlance of performance studies, Turner (1988, p. 42) holds that "cultural performances are reflective in the sense of showing ourselves to ourselves. They are also capable of being *reflexive*, arousing consciousness of ourselves as we see ourselves. As heroes in our own dramas, we are made self-aware, conscious of our own consciousness". The idea here is quite simple; if daily living is a kind of theatre, social drama is a kind of meta-theatre, that is, a dramaturgical language about the language of ordinary role-playing and status-maintenance which constitutes communication in the quotidian social process. In other words, when actors in a social drama try to show others what they are doing or have done, they are acting consciously, expressing *reflectiveness* or *reflexiveness*, the ability to communicate about the communication system it-self. This reflexivity is found not only in the eruptive phase of crisis, when one exerts one's wills and unleashes emotions to achieve one's goals, that is reflexivity following manifestation, but also in the cognitively dominant phase of redress where reflexivity is present from the outset, whether the redressive machinery is characterized as legal or ritual. The point to note here is with the process and processual qualities: performance, move, staging, plot, redressive action, crisis, schism, reintegration, and so on.

Furthermore, in the sense that man is a self-performing animal, Turner (1988, p. 8) posits that:

> ...his performances are, in a way, *reflexive*, in performing he reveals himself to himself. This can be in two ways: the actor may come to know himself better through acting or enactment; or one set of human beings may come to know themselves better through observing and/or participating in the performances generated and presented by another set of human beings. In the first instance, reflexivity is singular though enactment may be in a social context; in the second case, reflexivity is plural....

The major point to extrapolate from the above is that the basic thing about so-cial life is performance. The *self* is presented through the performance of roles, through performance that breaks roles, and through declaring to a given public that "one has undergone a transformation of state and status, been saved or damned, elevated or released" (Turner 1988, p. 81). In any case, social drama is a major form of plural reflexivity in a human social action. Plural reflexivity, as represented in the genres of performance differs from singular reflexivity in that it involves several persons in dramatic interaction. For instance, if there is a performance where a female performer dramatically stands her ground in a duel with her male counterpart and eventually floors him, then such a performance is not merely expressing the sheer willpower of one female and her ability to overcome, it is rather a philosophical statement challenging the patriarchal ori-entation and chauvinistic hegemony that has suppressed the women from time immemorial. It is indeed a total set of interactions which constitute this meta-commentary. This also explains what Schechner (1985, p. 35) calls "Restored Behaviour". Schechner contends that it is restored behaviour that is the main characteristic of performance. The practitioners of all these arts, rites, and healings assume that some behaviours, organized sequencesof events, scripted actions, known texts, scored movements, all exist separate from the performers who "do" these behaviours. This is because the behaviour is separate from those who are behaving, the behaviour can be stored, transmitted, manipulated, and transformed; the performers then get in touch with, recover, remember, or even invent these strips of behaviour and then "re-behave" according these strips either by being absorbed into them (i.e. playing the role, going into trance) or by existing side by side with them (as in the case of Brecht's "alienation effect"). Thus:

> ...restored behaviour is symbolic and reflexive... the self can act in/as another; the social or trans-individual self is a role or set of roles. Symbolic and reflexive behaviour is the hardening into theatre of social, religious, aesthetic, medical, and educational process. Performance means never for the first time. It means: for the second to the nth time. Performance is 'twice restored behaviour'. (Schechner 1985, p. 36)

The above being the case, the reflexive then becomes the responsibility of the performers and spectators alike, to not only recapitulate a sequence of events, but also to scrutinize and evaluate them. The re-enactment is framed as a performance, but it is actually a meta-performance, that is, a performance about a performance.

From the above exposition on the two strands of cultural performance theory selected for this study, it can be said that the concern with performance as a meaning-making communication system is common. If performance is the highest manifestation of culture as Fischer-Lichte reasons above, then cultural performance embodies and conveys the essence of culture, first to those who share it, and then to those who encounter it. In this study, for instance, reflexivity, which is concerned with self-awareness, self-consciousness, self-discovery, self-determination and so on, is relevant to the extent of understanding how the victims of the conflict under study show themselves to themselves and thereby arousing a consciousness of themselves as they see themselves reflected. The process of performance creation, staging, plotting redressive action, schism, reintegration, and so on all create a certain awareness that helps the communication of emotional information among people which leads to an overall healthier mental state. After all, individuals who experience strong social relationships have better overall health" (Bruhn 2005, p. 10). Thus, cultural performances would not only reflexively create a healthier mental state but also express and/or reflect the health of a society.

On the whole, performance theory is seen in this study as guiding the understanding of function and instrumentality of selected cultural performances under study; what they reflect, how they are perceived, the meaning they give, the power relations they communicate, the environment or atmosphere they create, their effectiveness in trauma management, their influence behavioural change, their capacity to collapse cultural binaries, and so on. This function and instrumentality will be closely viewed as it applies to the managing of collective trauma in victims of the farmers/herders' conflicts in Daudu Community.

2.7.2 Social Practice Theory

In other domains of sociology, particularly in relation to studies of consumption and sustainability, Shove (2003; 2007), Warde (2005) and others, have used social practice theories as developed by Schatzki (2001; 2002) and Reckwitz (2002; 2002) to broaden and enrich understandings of why people do what they do, and to offer alternative explanations of human 'action' other than behavioural understandings. In these post-humanist extensions of the theory, social practices are clearly the entity of study rather than individuals or their choices. There are three main features of theories of social practice as advanced in this, and other sustainability research, are broadly defined. Firstly, in post-humanist strains there is an emphasis on materiality whereby things, technologies and even infrastructures (Strengers and Maller 2012) are accounted for as active elements of practices with their own agency (Reckwitz 2002; Shove and Pantzar 2005).

Secondly, there is a clear distinction drawn between social practices as entities and social practices as performances, although the two are inherently bound together (Schatzki 1996; Warde 2005; Shove and Pantzar 2007). A practice as entity refers to the interrelated elements, or nexus, of a practice, as a recognisable 'doing' that is relatively stable (Schatzki 1996). Practice as performance describes the carrying out or performing of a practice, which ensures its continual reproduction (Schatzki 1996; Warde 2005; Shove and Pantzar 2007).

Thirdly, this distinction enables researchers to theorise about practice change, as it is through performance that practices evolve (Warde 2005; Shove and Pantzar 2007). In contrast, authors such as Frohlich et al (2001) comment that practice theory, or more specifically, Giddens' (1984) structuration theory, is said to struggle to account for change due to the mutually constitutive relationship between practices and wider social systems, which are difficult to separate and analyse independently. Using the distinction between entity and performance however, renders this theorisation possible. As Warde (2005,p. 141) explains, practices "contain the seeds of constant change… as people in myriad situations adapt, improvise and experiment". In this way, practices can be said to have 'trajectories' which are made up of minor modifications in past performances and the particular combination of elements at any one point in time (Warde 2005).

There is much more to elaborate on, particularly with regards to details about what contemporary strains of social practice theories can offer well-being research and how they improve upon predominant behavioural understandings. However, the above features of contemporary social practice theory bring to the study of health and well-being a clear way of acknowledging the materiality of spaces, places and things in everyday life, and understandings of how through performance and the incorporation of new elements into practice, daily routines may change over time.

In this study, the social practice theory is applied to anchor discussions that pertain to performance as a mechanism for managing collective trauma, and performance as a facilitator of cultural sustainability. The argument is that it is from continual practice that aspects of culture or everyday life find the guarantee that they may be relevant in the context of the future.

2.8 Conclusion

The literature reviewed in this chapter established perspectives on various conceptualisations and contexts that are of importance to this study. Prominent in this discourse is the conceptualisation of Procedural Sustainability which creates a unique nexus between the twin concerns of this study which bother on the question of cultural performance as a practice-based mechanism for managing collective trauma, and which practice also goes to enhance the possibility of same performances being available in the future – sustainability. The discourse on performance therapy and therapeutic performance also presented the dominant Western voice in the creative art therapies, a situation that suppresses or relegates the performative cultural practices in creative healing amongst non-Western societies. This is quite significant in this study as it directly links to a gap that studying cultural performances as a mechanism for managing collective trauma amongst displaced persons in Daudu Community aspires to contribute to filling. This is where the connection with cultural policy also finds a voice as such deliberate actions must be guided by tailored legal and operational frameworks that guide action from both state and non-state actors, hence the review of Nigeria's obsolete cultural policy document in line with international frameworks like the UNESCO 2005 Declaration on Cultural Diversity. The theories of cultural performance and social practice are espoused as guiding canons in the analysis of field data; whereas the cultural performance theory situates the aesthetic appreciation of the performances of the displaced to the extent of their form and function in managing collective trauma, the social practice theory anchors the argument that it is through practice that the performances will fulfil the role of helping the well-being of the displaced and at the same time remain available in the context of the future.

3 Methodology

The research methodology for this study is discussed under the following sub-headings: research design, study population and sample, research instruments, procedure for data collection, method of data analysis, and expected outcome. It is also important to note that this researcher is of the same ethnic group with the people of the study area, though not exactly from the same area of study. This situation offers an advantage for in-depth understanding of the content, nature and form of the cultural performances under study.

3.1 Research Design

The research adopted the qualitative methodology using the constructivist paradigm. It used the ethnographic approach to enable the researcher to systematically study the participants' viewpoint in natural contexts and provide a holistically participant informed perspective through what Geertz (1973) describes as "thick description" of cultural contexts. However, the study focused not only on participants' perception of cultural performances in the context of managing collective trauma, but also the integration of the richly described local cultural worlds in the larger complex of cultural sustainability. There was therefore a need for an approach that goes beyond the dominant descriptive ethnography often practiced, to an approach that penetrates hidden meanings and underlying connections. Critical ethnography, which is an ideologically sensitive orientation to the study of culture, was therefore applied as the preferred analytical approach as it is concerned with multiple perspectives, cultural and social inequalities and is directed towards positive social change. Performance ethnography, which exposes people of the same cultural contexts to performances and elicits their culture-based knowledge, understanding and experience of same is also critical to the analytical concerns of this study. Combining these approaches in this study availed the opportunity of achieving a more thorough understanding of the very complex nature of the social phenomena – cultural performances and collective trauma. This study is designed to explore the creative endeavours of the displaced persons which arose in the wake of these conflicts to tell their stories and deal with the traumatic experiences through songs, dance and dramatic enactments. The performances studied are those found within the community of the displaced population who performed for themselves and also utilized opportunities at public functions to communicate their experience and mobilise help.

3.2 Study Population and Sample

The population of this study is the entirety of the number of persons who have suffered in one way or the other in the wake of the perennial conflicts between farmers and herders in Benue State. The selected community of Daudu is in Guma LGA, twenty-two kilometres away from Makurdi, the Benue State capital. The people of Daudu are predominantly Tiv with a negligible mix of other ethnic nationalities occasioned by inter-tribal marriages and commerce. The language spoken in the community is Tiv. Largely, Daudu is a farming community with other sources of livelihoods such as trading, fishing and transportation.

Indeed, it can be said that the entire Benue population has suffered from these conflicts, either directly or indirectly. Direct victims are therefore those who have suffered horrendous experiences including bodily harm, loss of property, livelihoods and relations; whereas the indirect victims are those who have to endure social and psychological stress arising from panic, accommodation of direct victims, sharing of resources with direct victims, and the general discomfort arising from the actual presence of direct victims in the community of the consciousness of having 'displaced persons' around. The population of Benue State is approximated at 4.3 million people while that of Guma LGA where Daudu is located is 191,599 (National Population Commission, 2006). Daudu itself is a town with estimated population of 4,000 people. Since qualitative research designs focus less on a sample's representativeness or on detailed techniques for drawing a probability sample (Neuman, 2009), but rather on how the small sample or small collection of cases, units, or activities, illuminates social life or the phenomenon being studied, the primary purpose of sampling in this study is to collect specific cases, or actions that can clarify or deepen the researcher's understanding about the phenomenon under study, which is the effect of cultural performances in managing collective trauma amongst displaced victims of farmers/herders conflicts in Benue State. Effectively therefore, this study was based on the conduct of five Key Informant Interviews (KII), two Focus Group Discussions (FGDs) comprising eight group members, several observation field trips to the camps and other places where the population is found, and observation of population in performance ethnography sessions.

3.3 Data Collection Methods

The study employed the following qualitative methods for data gathering:

1. **Key Informant Interview (KII):** For this study, the key informants were carefully selected to reflect informants who have first-hand knowledge about the case study community, its residents, and issues or problems surrounding the farmers/herders conflicts, and the pertinence of art-based approaches to peace and healing. Community members knowledgeable in the cultural ways of the people were also specifically targeted. The fifteen key informants targeted for this study were drawn from a variegated range including agency representatives, arts professionals, psychologists, community residents, community leaders, church leaders, neighbourhood-watch-association representatives, parents, youth advocates, and the police. This diversity was to provide a broad range of perspectives.
2. **Focus Group Discussion:** For this study, two focus groups of eight members were carried out. Since the population is homogenous and the questions simple, meaning saturation was easily reached.
3. **The Performances:** the cultural performances amongst the study population themselves are an instrument for data collection. The people were observed in the performance sessions and further discussions about the performances done with groups. This helped in providing additional insight into the experience of the people as the instances they encountered were reproduced in these performances.
4. **Participant Observation:** the researcher observed to make a reflection and isolate salient issues that did not necessarily form part of the interviews and focus group discussions from amongst the study subjects, but were quite germane to the thrust of the study. Video recordings were also made during field engagements and they also provided the researcher the opportunity for further observation and reflection. The researcher also actively participated in some singing and dancing sessions.

3.4 Procedure for Data Collection

In pursuit of data gathering for this study, the researcher relied on his earlier established contacts while working for a non-governmental organization (Foundation for Justice, Peace and Development, Makurdi) which was promoting peacebuilding initiatives in the community. This facilitated access to community and statutory set ups. This earlier established relationship was equally important with regards to wadding off suspicions that would have arisen from prospective study subjects leading to a withholding of information. Three research assistants were engaged, one of which was female. The assistants were trained on the nature of data sought, recording and note-taking skills and interpersonal relationship skills with study subject. Key informant interviews were conducted first and information gathered therefrom was cross checked at the FGD. Issues raised from both the KII and FGD formed the basis for observation in order to ascertain whether these performances have significant impact on the recovery process of the displaced persons who are victims of farmers/herders conflicts in Daudu Community. Data gathered was analysed for purposes of writing the final report.

3.5 Method of Data Analysis

The basic activity in the analysis of data generated in this study was reading of texts, notes, transcripts, documents and listening or viewing audio and video materials. It is important to note that the term "text" as used here embraces not just printed material, but also pictures, posters, recorded music, film and television. In fact, any cultural product can be read as text. Thus, the reading of texts here was done in the light of the research questions including those which arose during the data collection process.

3.6 Validity and Reliability

The validity and reliability of a qualitative study is ensured by applying the key principles of rigour/trustworthiness. Reliability denotes the "stability of research results and their ability to be replicated" and validity involves "whether or not researchers have actually discovered what they claim to have found, and the extent to which what they have learned can be applied to other populations" (Schensul, & LeCompte, 1999, p. 271). Thus, studies that fail to observe rigour result in several problems; as such, the results cannot be trusted and the understanding of the phenomenon becomes blurred (Cho & Trent, 2006).

Ethnographers over the years have debated issues of validity and reliability because the principles and practice of ethnography as in data collection and analysis do not lend themselves to the positivists' emphasis on control that is used to describe principles of validity and reliability. It is recognized that the subjective perspective of the researcher during ethnographic data collection and analysis and the naturalistic nature of data collection superimposes the "control" in experimental studies. Therefore, the implementation of standard principles of validity and reliability becomes problematic in ethnographic studies (LeCompte &

Schensul, 1999b; Parahoo, 2006; Patton, 1999). This study holds that all studies must ensure the necessary rigour rather than a researcher being preoccupied with terminologies used to describe rigorous processes. Researchers should endeavour to adopt the appropriate techniques based on the type of study to ensure that findings that emanate from the study can be appreciated within a particular paradigm.

Thus, this study identifies with Patton, (1999) that credibility of qualitative research depends on rigorous techniques and methods during data collection and analysis, the credibility of the researcher based on training and experience, and the philosophical belief in the value of enquiry. Strategies that are employed to achieve rigour of a particular study depend on the design of the study and the applicability of the strategy. Thus, researchers should be circumspect in their choice of strategies to ensure rigour. Based on the foregoing argument therefore, the ethnographic explorative phase of this study employed the following strategies to ensure rigour:

3.6.1 Multiple Data Collection Methods

Methodological triangulation in this study involved several data collection methods such as interviews, participant observation, focus group discussions, performance ethnography and video recording review to enable the researcher to answer the research question. The use of several data collection methods in a particular study is believed to provide a broader perspective than the use of a single method of data collection (LeCompte & Schensul, 1999b; Saks &Allsop, 2007). The researcher is aware that the use of several data collection methods does not guarantee validity of findings; but, rather it is the ability to ensure that all the data collection methods used maintain the required standards (Parahoo, 2006) that counts. In this study therefore, the use of multiple data collection enhanced the credibility of results.

3.6.2 Member-Checks

This is also known as participant validation; and involves going back to informants with transcripts and/or data analysis so that they can confirm, or repudiate the researcher's conclusions. Participant validation is seen to offer participants some form of involvement in the study and also provides the researcher an opportunity to reconsider the interpretation of the data based on a constructive discussion during member checking. The process of member checking ensures that the *emic* perspective is highlighted and represented "truthfully". The insight gained from previous authors on participant validation provided the confidence for this researcher that the use of member checking in this study to ensure rigor is creditable. Therefore, feedback discussions were held within the community of the displaced persons and it was open to participants beyond those in the earlier FGD sessions to ensure validity. A performance ethnography was carried out and themes discussed with everyone present given the opportunity to voice their feelings about the identified themes in the performances.

3.7 Ethical Considerations

The researcher is obliged to maintain high ethical standards during a particular study. Thus, permission was sought from the gatekeepers within the Daudu Community involved with the IDP situation. The researcher negotiated for access to the camp and its surroundings at any time and on any day to ensure full access to the study setting. After obtaining approval from the gatekeepers, consent was sought from the individual participants before they were engaged in the study activities. Specific ethical principles employed are explained below.

3.7.1 Participant Language

Most of the field activities were conducted in Tiv language so as to ensure that participants clearly understood every step of the activities and could freely express themselves more conveniently. Some in-depth interviews were conducted in English language. The researcher also has mastery of the Tiv language and therefore it was easy to ensure that participants described their world articulately and the understanding of same was based on their context.

The use of participant language is also known as thick descriptions in qualitative research where the researcher uses verbatim quotations of the participants' words in the research report. The use of participants' culturally specific terms or words is to give the reader an insight into the participants' world. The contextual description and the researcher's interpretation of these verbatim quotes help in the transferability of ethnographic studies; whereby the reader is able to compare findings to similar context. Also, native languages cited as verbatim quotes in the research report are translated to afford an understanding of the participants' comments (Atkinson and Hammersley, 1994; LeCompte & Schensul, 1999b; Patton, 2002) and these principles were applied in this thesis.

3.7.2 Informed Consent

The researcher had discussions with the Benue State Emergency Management Agency in-charge of the IDP situation and also the leadership in the camp. The general camp population were also made aware of the research activities and the consent to observe their lives and hold talks with them. The right to withdraw from the study at any time was also explained. Further clarifications were given on data protection where it was stressed that if they were not comfortable with being recorded or their shared opinions being divulged they could say so and this will be highly respected. The participants were unanimous that they have nothing to hide as long as the purposes of the study remain to understand their situation and communicate same to the wider world. All methods/processes of data collection were explained such as participant observation, review of video recordings/notes, and individual interviews. Participants were informed about note-taking during observations and recording interviews with an audio recorder. Stakeholders and experts involved in the in-depth interviews also gave consent in this study and the permission to quote them directly.

3.8 Data Management

Interviews were recorded with a digital voice recorder which allowed for transfer of recorded voice files onto a personal computer. Interviews were transcribed in the language they were conducted, which were Tiv and English languages. In the interpretation and discussion of findings where translation is done of responses in Tiv language, focus was strictly on the meaning of the participant's contribution and those conducted in English were transcribed verbatim.

3.9 Researcher Positionality

In qualitative research and in ethnographic studies, the researcher is the primary research instrument. In this thesis, the researcher's background and interest in this study is provided. It is recognized that the researcher's personal, professional or disciplinary biases and perspectives affect the research questions, data collection and analysis, and how the findings are interpreted (Schensul et al., 1999; Smith, 1996; Spradley, 1979b). It is therefore necessary to report the researcher's reflections on his role as a performer-researcher and a member of the Tiv ethnic nationality who form the majority of displaced farmer communities in Benue State.

The advantage of being a performer-researcher and a member of the ethnic nationality are twofold. As a performer-researcher, it was easy to connect to the performance context within which the displaced persons express themselves. This also made it easy to probe further on the meanings and experiences of the people within disciplinary peculiarities in Performance Studies. Also, as a member of the ethnic stock, it was easier for the participants to trust the researcher with their experiences and bare their minds without any reservations. The medium of communication was also very convenient because both researcher and participants did not have language barriers and this made mutual understanding very easy.

It is important to state also that the motivation for this was born out of the researcher's everyday encounter with the traumatic experiences of displaced persons and the burning desire to do something about the situation. Several interventions from state and non-state actors have been going on in the wake of the violent relations between farmers and herders but a resolution of the conflict does not seem to be in sight. Rather, masses of displaced person increase and the squalid conditions of the camps in which they are forced to live in further compounds their trauma. This research project became compelling out of the need to find cultural approaches that are readily available to the people and do not require specialised training to help in the management of the collective trauma they experience. The idea is to find out how viable the cultural performance mechanism is in managing trauma amongst the displaced persons so that civil society organizations, faith-based organizations, community leaders and state actors could begin to pay more serious attention to these cultural approaches, and the people themselves will become bold and more trusting in this approach as being quintessential in negotiating a more meaningful vision for their lives and out of their prevailing state of helplessness and hopelessness.

It is however important to state that my positionality did not interfere with the objectivity of data gathered and the analysis of same. For instance, the participants in the FGD session could confidently share information and opinion about herders where they said not all of them are bad as some of them are sympathetic of their plight and also yearn for the cordial relationship that existed between them before the hostilities.

3.10 Conclusion

This chapter discussed the appropriateness of a qualitative approach and hence the application of the principles of ethnography to the study in contrast with other qualitative methods. The chapter also described the design adopted for the study. The chapter described the context or location of the study, and the population and the rationale for the choice of the population. The issues of rigour in this study were also discussed in-depth and the data analysis strategies were described. The chapter ended with a highlight on the impact of the researcher's positionality on the study.

4 The Cultural Performances

This chapter presents the findings of this study based on data generated and analysed. It is divided into three main sections. The first section presents the nature and form of cultural performances as found amongst the internally displaced persons in Daudu Community; this includes their music, their dances and their dramatic enactments. Cultural performances as explored in this segment are as performed by the displaced people within the Daudu Community, Benue State, Nigeria, and this means that there is also a cultural context within which these performances exist and are appreciated. Considering that the displaced population under study homogenously comes from the same ethnic nationality, the Tiv, it is pertinent to examine the nature of cultural performances amongst the Tiv. This will then form the background against which the folk songs, dance/movement, and dramatic enactments as experienced amongst the displaced persons in Daudu, in the context of collective trauma management are explored. The second section is dedicated to the contextual findings on the research questions based on the ethnographic exploration involving the displaced persons, civil society workers, academics and a clinical psychologist. The third section presents findings from the systematic review of literature (secondary data), highlighting recommended measures in the current evidence on cultural performances and collective trauma that can be applied in the context of this study and thus providing the basis for the new perspective to be properly situated.

4.1 Cultural Performances amongst the Tiv

Despite the influence of other cultures, especially those of the West, with attendant factors such as globalisation and Christianity, the Tiv people have retained a dense cultural heritage as an important asset that arguably makes them popular across cultures within Nigeria and beyond. This, perhaps may explain why different nationalities and groups admire and adorn Tiv dresses, savour Tiv music, and appreciate their language, literature and art. Tiv warfare, occupation and trade, marriage practices, social and covenantal relations and history are also cultural items which other cultures and groups talk about with relish (Andera 2015). According to Akpede (2010, p. 6), "Tiv performing arts originate from music, singing, and dancing or sound and movement... (and) these performances are in unlimited variations". It is true that Tiv performances are unlimited in their variations, but what may be misleading in the above postulation by Akpede is the claim that Tiv performing arts "originate" from the mentioned arts; it is rather more accurate to say that the mentioned arts are forms of Tiv performing arts since the origins of most indigenous performances are lost in prehistory. It is therefore safer to rely on Ogunbiyi's (1981) submission that all the performances of the different Nigerian ethnic groups originate from the religious and secular festivals of the different Nigerian ethnic groups. As one of the dominant ethnic groups, those of the Tiv too must have derived from similar sources.

On another count, it is pertinent to note that many of Tiv dances are vigorous, energy sapping and enduring, and are products of particular periods and social experience. There are however dance styles associated with the advanced in age, these styles are collectively known as *Uzagigh* meaning the aged. Such styles are slow, lacking in energy but indeed graceful. As a matter of fact, there is no serious Tiv gathering that is devoid of music, songs and dances, which are no doubt the most commonly used in every Tiv festival performance or other social function. The reason is simple: they create entertainment and recreation, and at the same time communicate through possible bodily exhibition in form of movement, through mime and pantomimic dramatization so as to pass a message, consciously or unconsciously to the audience who are most times caught in as participants. In buttressing the fact that there is no occasion that lacks dance of whatever kind amongst the Tiv, Ahura succinctly posits that "music and dance are so central to Tiv life that even the Tiv market which should be a place for economic activities is usually turned into an arena for showbiz, making a strong point about the connection between dance, music, economy and politics" (p.16). This is true for most Tiv markets, dance and music feature freely. If one goes to most Tiv markets, one discovers that these activities are interwoven and juxtaposed with the business activities which are supposed to be the mainstay of such markets. Ahura's position has gone ahead to confirm the fact that dance is part of the socio-cultural and economic life of the people which has been passed down from generation to generation. Andera (2015) takes the argument further to posit that "other than markets, political gatherings which have become popular nowadays equally attract different categories of artistes from singers to dancers. All these throng the political assembly to entertain guests and help disseminate the manifesto of the party as well as to ridicule members of rival political parties" (p.8). The idea from the forgoing argument is that whatever the nature of the occasion, performances of various kinds are done either to entertain, educate and sensitize the participating audience.

Considering the significance of these arts to the Tiv people, it is expedient to state that the folktales are basically didactic in nature and are used in sharpening and shaping the young minds intellectually, and schooling them in societal norms and values. Ahura, again, cogently argues that"

> ...the central function of the tales is to help in ensuring egalitarianism and fairness in the society. People who try to move away from the communal norms in order to assert their individuality are roundly chastised and corrected through examples of similar characters in the folktales while those who work for the good of the community are valorised. (p.124)

The thrust of the above is to buttress the egalitarian ethos in Tiv folktales. Towards this end, the tales help to entrench the egalitarian nature of the Tiv society and also teach members to imbibe communal living as opposed to individualism.

The song composers (who are almost always also the performers) on their part assert the solidarity of their own group and at the same time recognize their close relationship with others. The songs may even provide a means for psychological release of repressed enmities and tensions through a socially permissible form. Festivals on the other hand serve as a means through which the Tiv appease their gods. The traditional or cultural dances that emanate from these ritualistic festivities serve the purpose of communal expression of emotions which lie beyond ordinary speech. Quite significantly, it is incumbent upon performing artists, having enjoyed the acceptability and patronage of society, to imbue an awakening of cultural consciousness and engender social reform where there are observations on culturally conflicting phenomena, a call for something better, and the urge to setup models for the society of the future. Such awakening of consciousness as mentioned here often makes for solidarity with the past, which does not however hamper progressive innovation, but rather function as a vehicle for resisting all that threaten the social cohesiveness of the group. Generally, Tiv cultural performances act in response to the collective yearnings, aspiration and solicitations of the people; this function becomes even more incumbent as a demonstration of the strength and steadfastness in the face of anything that threatens their culture's primordial originality. This is also perceived as the same reason for the systematization and regularization of traditional festivals amongst the various communities across the African continent. This cannot be far from the truth since the festival is the only traditional institution which can coordinate all the arts of a community. In the process of performance, the arts of costuming, masking, chanting, singing, dancing, acting, miming, drumming, and several other aspects of performing arts are served. These performances evoke history and age-long artistic forms of the community, and galvanise the people into envisaging a common future that they collectively work towards.

From the foregoing discourse therefore, it is appropriate for one to posit that Tiv performing arts are holistically a reflection and expression of Tiv worldview and cosmology. The different art forms express their hopes and fears, successes and failures, toils and moils, as well as explain their interactions with their natural environment. Through these performances, the Tiv regulate and maintain their world. Through the same medium, cultural aspects are transmitted from generation to generation.

Like elsewhere, Tiv traditional performances can be sacred and secular considering the functions they fulfil in socio-religious context. Basically, these performances are rooted in the Tiv culture, and because of this, the people are continually creating works of art which tend to offer a deep appraisal of their actions, their hopes, frustrations and their achievements. Uji (1993) avers that "there are several genres of Tiv performing arts…these include the folktale, riddle, song, dance, music and the *Kwagh-hir*" (51). In any case, performances such as the *Kwagh-hir*, certain social dances like *Swange, Gberichul, Ihinga*, and the comic forms are devoid of ritualism hence secular, whereas those with ritual elements of worship and propitiation like *Ivom, Iee, Igbe, Ibiamegh, Girinya*, and so on are considered sacred.

Quite significantly, cultural performances of the Tiv reflect their customs, values, and belief system which operate to teach and mould a strong Tiv community and their worldview. Hagher (1987) captures this functional pre-occupation of the Tiv cultural performances well when he submits that "The Tiv traditional theatre exhibits curious traits that combine the theatre of totality as well as a total theatre in a synthesis that is more than human, ritualistic, ironic and heretic as opposed to the traditional popular Western theatre" (p. 6). Gbilekaa (1993) corroborates this standpoint when he succinctly avers that "The Tiv man gives more attention to serious and philosophical aspects of life believing that no sane and serious man would delve into banal, impious and non-serious aspects of life unmasking them through action" (p. 4). This postulation is a confirmation that the Tiv cultural performances, like other African theatre types, are not a mere presentation of dramatic episodes but a presentation that is functionally dynamic.

In all the genres, one observes that all principles of aesthetic design like harmony, rhythm, variety, grace, unity, precision, emphasis, balance, and proportion are greatly underscored within their body politic. This means that all the components of the particular genre in question have to congruously combine and lead to the complete realization of its thematic pre-occupation. For example, a song which functions as a dirge, of necessity must organically have its parts arranged in such a way that the resultant mood and the central message depict mourning. However, this does not suggest that all Tiv songs have a monolithic theme. In fact, many of them engross a variety of important themes; what the principle insists upon is that each theme should be appropriately realized by the proper fusion of the parts.

In addition, the didacticism of Tiv cultural performances is one other area deserving significance mention. This principle is all-embracing in its manifestation in that it embodies history, ethics, politics, religion, and education, among other existential concerns. This principle makes clear the fact that aestheticism in Tiv arts has a strong functionalist base, and that it is consciously didactic in its consideration of form and content. It is very usual amongst responsible and critical Tiv audiences, after a performance, to pose questions such as: what particular lesson is the show trying to teach? Apparently, if such a show lacks an articulate pedagogical message, it is generally considered as irrelevant because the profundity of form is expected to match that of content.

Furthermore, one other general aesthetic principle that cuts across all the genres is decorum which detests in unmitigated terms the issue of pornography in art. In this light, Uji (1993) posits that "pornographic songs and dances, for instance, are considered bohemian and their audience is usually comprised of maladroit and morally decadent members of the society like prostitutes and their male patrons" (p. 51). Examples of this sort include *kpingi* and *ngigh-ngigh*, which properly speaking do not belong to the Tiv aesthetic canon. In present times, those who patronize such performances do so under the cover of dark; the performances are usually offered at night and in poor lit spaces because of the indecency they connote and no one wants to be associated with that.

Nevertheless, as true as it is that the very principles as outlined here traverse all the genres of Tiv cultural performances, it is very instructive to understand that some are specifically peculiar to certain genres especially from the perspective of form. The essentially verbal arts, like the folktale and the song, have a propensity for the creative use of proverbs, allusions, personifications, repetitions and hyperboles in their form and structure. In performance, for example, dance demands the flexible use of the entire body to achieve aesthetic communication with the aid of appropriate costume, makeup and other relevant histrionic accessories.

Cultural performance amongst the Tiv comprises a total experience that features a variety of theatrical elements in a given performance. This implies that in a given performance, there is the interplay of different theatrical elements in order to realize a satisfying performative experience. Some of these elements such as gestures, facial expressions, space, body movement, design and music are devoid of words; they are realized through non-verbal communication, yet they are quite important because they contribute to the understanding of the performances. To understand these performances, it behoves the audience to possess good cultural knowledge of non-verbal communication, since much of the meaning in these performances is embedded in the cultural context of these non-verbal cues which could be gestures, symbols, costumes, signs and even make up. These non-verbal codes are numerous and are used in ordinary day interaction with fellow beings, and also come handy either while acting in the conventional theatre or in traditional African performances. In all situations, they aim to aid the audience to make meaning in the communication process as humans beings make use of these either consciously or unconsciously to put across messages. These actions individually and collectively make definite statements about the state and feeling of the speaker's sex, socio-economic status, political affiliation, religious group and level of educational attainment. These signs and images are important in appreciating Tiv cultural performances. Extrapolating on this, Doki (2006, p. 66) avers that Tiv performances...

> ...employ(s) a lot of signs and imagery in communication. Language, movement, acting, costume, staging techniques, colours, lighting and characterization used in performances hold deep forms or greater values in terms of structure and meaning. They are signs, which are symbolic and in fact, explain the need for the performance as well as situate man in relation with the cosmic.

It therefore follows that where one does not understand them, one does not stand the chance of understanding these performances.

On the whole, the Tiv in their cultural performances employ numerous theatrics all at the service of a particular function – social reengineering. The songs with their didactic lessons, the *Kwagh-hir* which lampoons the society and projects the ideal, the dances which entertain and communicate cosmological permutations and implications, and the other forms all co-exist to fulfil this onerous role. The cultural performances are about what the people know, have experienced, do and are familiar with. They serve as a reservoir of the people's culture, arts, and beliefs, religious and even architectural designs. The idea is that there is no room for art for art's sake in both the sacred and secular spheres; whether the performance elements occur in singular or collective forms, the aim is uniquely singular.

4.2 Cultural Performances by the Displaced Persons in Daudu Community

The displaced persons in Daudu Community do not claim to be of an ethnic extraction other than the Tiv, whose performance traditions are significantly discussed above. Thus, the performances found amongst the displaced population in the study community are the same with those described above in terms of nature, form, structure, and cultural aesthetics. However, the thematic preoccupation, and indeed the aesthetic accompaniments of performances within the community of the displaced are unique to the extent of their context of operation. The performances are either an adaptation of old forms of cultural enactments to suit their present reality, or some improvisation sufficient for aesthetic functionalism.

In buttressing the fact that Tiv people are culturally a performative people, who like to tell their stories through songs, music and dance, and are quick to finding ways of redefining their events and moments through arts, Tor Iorapuu (personal communication, 16 March, 2019) posits that "if you take the '*Ingyôugh*' dance for instance, it is another performative experience that tries to depict various illnesses that had befallen the people … so the Tiv people through '*Kwagh-hir*' and through dance, and other narrative performances try to tell their story". Iorapuu (personal communication, 16 March, 2019) goes ahead to submit that the experience from the displaced persons

> …is even more unique in the sense that we have a situation here where the people themselves are frustrated, nobody is coming to their aid, nobody is listening to them, so they have to find a creative way of letting people hear them directly, because often times when other people speak to them, the reality, you know, their traumatic experiences are not captured as deep as they would do it themselves.

The idea here is that the displaced persons come from a culturally creative and artistically expressive stock and therefore are quick to resort to a mechanism that is already embedded in them.

The place of improvisation and spontaneity in the performances of the displaced is quite central and critical. Though definitions vary, improvisation is most often described as a process of "making it up as you go along" (Harlpen, Close and Johnson 1994), though, ironically, this ability to be creative is premised on highly repetitive exercises, processes and protocols that enable students to develop the skills to be creative in their response to new scenarios or situation. In theatrical contexts, then, making it up as you go along does not necessarily mean anything goes. Making it up as you go along more typically means applying rules, routines or response possibilities/processes practiced over time to a new scenario, a new set of hurdles, in a spontaneous and creative way. It combines convergent and divergent thinking, repetitive and creative processes, openness and play with clear, goal-directed action. This is a valuable skill. It helps us negotiate a landscape, learn, and come up with new ideas. It helps us manage our own actions. It helps us manipulate our interactions with others. All of which is highly advantageous in adapting as a given story, scenario or situation plays out, whether in dramatic performance, or in day-to-day performance in social contexts.

It is important to note, as experienced with the performances of the displaced persons that grotesque and frightening things are released as soon as people begin to work with spontaneity (Johnson 1989), and spontaneity means abandoning some of your defences. Improvisation has long been recognised as useful in teaching children to cope with their world, in community work, and in therapy, as well as in coming up with characters, scenes, stories and insight in an actor training or theatrical context.

In contrast, improvisational theatre has no script and no memorized lines or actions. Actors "write" and perform scenes simultaneously. They do so spontaneously and collaboratively. They create and develop their characters in the same manner. Actors often mime or otherwise suggest aspects of the environment, which the audience experiences through their shared imagination. A common misconception is that "anything goes" in improvisation. For some, to suggest an improvisational approach implies anarchy, such assumptions obscure understanding and can be prejudicial. The fact is: "Improvisation, although it involves spontaneity and extemporizing, doesn't mean that there is a total lack of structure" (Sawyer 2000). Weick (1998) explained that "you can't improvise on nothing; you've gotta improvise on something". Structure is important in improvisation, though it may not be obvious to an audience. Structure provides a framework for improvisation, and in this case, it is the prevalent performance structure from the cultural background of the people that manifests. Improvisation amongst the displaced is prevalent in all their performances; from the songs which are full of instantaneous adlibs, through sudden gestures in the dance movements to the unstructured nature of the dramatic enactments wherein each participant is free and welcome to introduce an element based on a particular experience in their flight from violence or the uncomfortable living conditions they are under. These are circumstances they have all come to share and are therefore able to relate with immediately whenever such an experience is introduced into the dramatic performances at whatever point.

One other characteristic of these performances is their interconnectedness even though one can still identify them by their distinct individual forms. Movement is central and common to the individually identifiable forms of Music, Dance and Drama. Musicking here requires movement; in fact making music in the African context is singing, instrumentation, rhythm, and movement all combined. Dance is basically rhythmic movement within time and space and drama also requires movement to execute action. One therefore finds an interaction of these performance forms that revolves around movement which must deliberate, purposeful, motivated, characteristic, simplified, and in some instances heightened.

It can be noticed from the above illustration that there is an interconnection between one form and another before the central point which connects all forms as movement. African dance involves drama enactments, African drama encompasses dance elements, African music compels dance and dramatisation and so on. This means that dance and music can interact independently just as drama and music or dance and drama, but the overall denominator in the entire matrix remains creative movement.

4.2.1 Music: Folk Songs

The Tiv people find it very easy to express themselves through singing. Indeed, music and dance are so central to Tiv life that every aspect of their socio-cultural and economic life is laced with it. Perhaps this is why the most dominant genre of the cultural performances even amongst the displaced persons is the song mode.

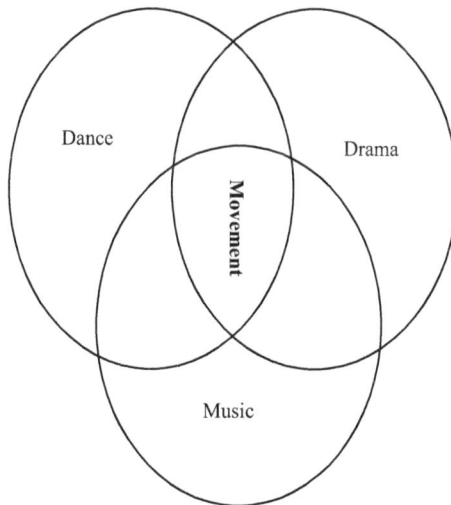

Fig. 1: The Ukuma Illustration on Interconnectivity of African Dance, Drama and Music

Music as experienced in this context is devoid of instrumentation, except for clapping of hands or tapping of feet. As the songs flow, a general rhythm is established and this determines the pace of performance. The composition of the songs is equally simple with short verses which are basically in the form of call and response. There is usually a verse and a chorus to which the crowd responds. The lead singer, who has to be the most skilled at voice dynamics or the next most skilled and in that order, takes the verse at the end of which the crowd responds with the chorus. This creates an engaging atmosphere and enhances group participation. Each time the lead singer takes the verse, she is likely to (and she usually does) introduce critical elements into the lyrics so as to deepen the message; new names of persons and places are introduced, new experiences or encounters with violence are narrated, and things like that.

Numerous songs were encountered and collected in the course of the fieldwork. However, a careful review and observation of these songs in performance helped the researcher to narrow down to six songs which are analysed below. These six songs stood out as they created a more engaging atmosphere for a generality of the displaced persons to participate. The songs carry a more holistic picture of their experiences and they have in them more performative nuances that spur the people more into expressive actions.

Song One

Tiv	English
Oo imbya ne mba er nena?	Oh! What's done in a matter as this?
On-Tiv oo imbya ne mba er nena o,	Tiv offspring, what's done in a
Oo imbya mba er nena?	matter as this?
Agwei zenda Tiv oo, imbya mba	Oh! What's done in a matter as this?
er nena	*Agwei* has sent away the Tiv oo,
On-Tiv oo imbya mba er nena? (2x)	what's done in a matter as this?
	Tiv offspring, what's done in a
	matter as this?

In this song, the displaced sing about the general sense of disorientation and helplessness. In the song, the displaced do not seem to know what to do in their volatile circumstances, thus they ask "what's done in a matter as this?" They address their question to the younger and more energetic youths whom they consider as more knowledgeable in the circumstance and who perhaps would be more proactive to address their woes. The song also makes a sweeping accusation

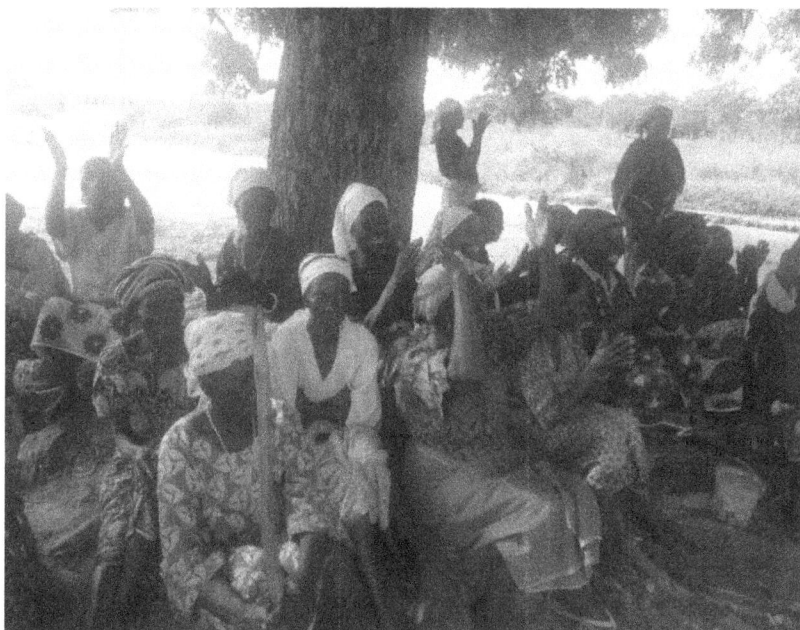

Plate 1: Displaced Women at a Singing session (Ukuma 2018)

that the "*Agwei*" (a local nickname for the Fulani herder) has ransacked the Tiv, meaning also that it is the entire Tiv nation that has been attacked. This conveys collective victimhood and at the same time wins over into sympathy Tiv or their friends who may feel safe since they may not be experiencing any physical attack themselves. This, to an extent also implicates all those who in one way or the other could do something to salvage their conditions. The song is also silent about any provocations or retaliations, but rather focuses on the concern for a way out of the circumstances.

In a focus group discussion session, the participants specifically articulated that their song performances are lamentations unto their children and others who could help:

Agwei ngu a zenda u we a za gba shighen u genegh u ndivir, nyityô kwagh i genegh jSe kpaa i fatyô u eren we her. Ve se lu vaan mlyam man se aluer se alu a mbayev kera yô, ve ungwa mlyam ma ujija mba ungôôv vev mban ve lu vaan ne.
Mlyam ma se lu vaan man ka sha ci u mbavesen mbara ve ungwa kwagh u Fulani ve lu eren a vese ne. (FGD 2018)

When the *Agwei* (herders) chase after you and you fall, sometimes you dislocate, any other thing at all could happen to you there. That is why we cry out so that if at all we have children out there, let them hear the cry that their old broken mothers are crying.
The lamentation (referring to songs) we do is such that the big people (those in authority) should hear what the Fulani are doing to us. (FGD, St. Francis Mission, Daudu 2018)

The notion as expressed in the excerpt above presents the essence of the singing endeavour. The displaced persons are convinced that help has to come, but they must also reach out to the world in order to tell by themselves what the challenge is, and also take responsibility in asking for help.

Song 2

TIV	ENGLISH
A hia kpa a hia wan mbaior	If they're burnt they should burn; child of a people
Akôr a hia kpa a hia ka uma wase ga	If the yam-seedlings are burnt they should burn, it's not our lives
A hia kpa a hia wan mbaior	If they're burnt they should burn; child of a people
Akôr a hia kpa a hia ka uma wase ga	If the yam-seedlings are burnt they should burn, it's not our lives
Alôgô rumun zwa wase ga,	The Alôgô[2] do not accept our tribe
Torkula Fulani rumun zwa wase ga	Torkula[3] Fulani do not accept our tribe
Ior mban zua zwa a vese m kar ayem o	These people have ganged up against us, I'm on the run
Akôr a hia kpa a hia ka uma wase ga	If the yam-seedlings are burnt they should burn, it's not our lives

In Song 2, the general message is about the value the displaced attach to their lives above material things and properties. In this song, the displaced people dismiss with outright nonchalance their burnt yam-seedlings, and by extension their entire crops and livelihoods, saying that those things are not their lives, meaning it is more important to them to be alive.

The song also articulates the perceived conspiracy against the Tiv ethnic group by their neighbours, the Arago (pronounced *Alôgô* by the Tiv) and the Fulani to whom the Arago have been a long time vassal. In the song, the displaced performers go further to petition to Torkula, the then king of the Tiv people

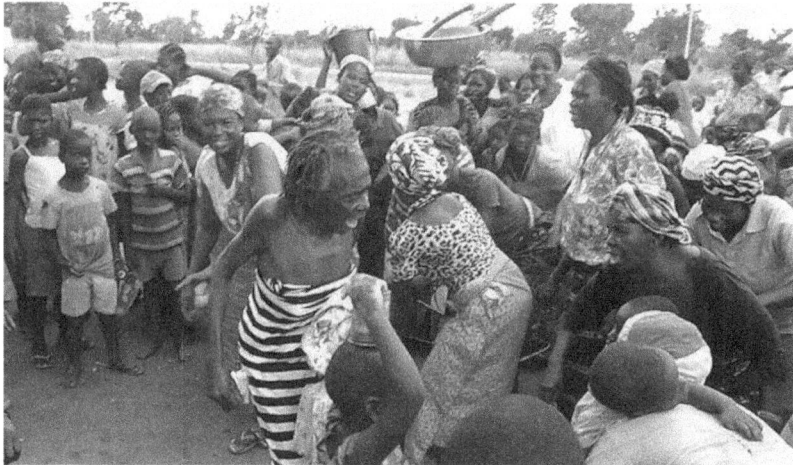

Plate 2: The displaced persons pictured here dancing. The bending posture here communicates how they duck from the weapons of their assailants (Ukuma 2018)

that the Fulani and Arago do not like their tribe and have thus conspired against them that is why they are on the run.

Song 3

Tiv	English
Se se vaa alôm ô	We hole-up like the hare
Se se vaa alôm ô (2x)	We hole up like the hare (2x)
Or Agwei zungul aga kerem ve oo	The *Agwei* flung his ox-goad at me oo
Aga tam veoo or Agwei wuam aa (2x)	The ox-goad has hit me oo, the *Agwei* has killed me

Song three is a narration of assailing action of the marauding herders. The song talks about the herder swinging his ox-goad at the fleeing farmers who then duck and hole up like a rabbit. This describes actions of attack and the evasive tactics of the farmer communities. The ox-goad is used in the song to represent every form of weapon used, and the choice is because it symbolically represents the herders.

Song 4

TIV	ENGLISH
Ve tim Ihyarev gba gban bee ee	They've annihilated the *Ihyarev*, so vast and severe
On tim Ihyarev gba gban bee ee	They've annihilated the *Ihyarev*, so vast and severe
Or u Mbalam karem a wan sha (2x)	Man of *Mbalam*⁴ go away with my child (2x)
Or u Mbalam karem a wan	Man of *Mbalam* go away with my child
On tim Ihyarev gba gban bee ee	They've annihilated the *Ihyarev*, so vast and severe

The theme in song four is annihilation and safety for the children. The song tells of the vast and severe destruction of the *Ihyarev* sub-area of the Tiv people. Indeed this area is the worst hit in the conflict situation and the community where this study is carried out is located within this sub-area.

The concern for the safety of children is expressed in the song where "Man of *Mbalam*" (*Mbalam* being a further sub-clan of the *Ihyarev*) is asked to go away with the children. The song calls out to the "man" because of the Tiv cosmological

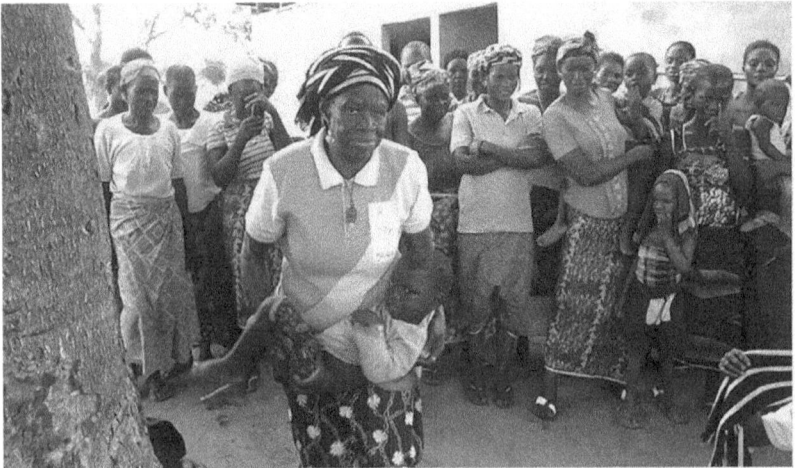

Plate 3: A woman is pictured here carrying a child to safety (Ukuma 2018)

notion that wars are affairs of men so to evacuate people and property in front-line areas is a masculine task.

Song 5

TIV	ENGLISH
Ôn-Tiv oo! Ne ne ungwa kwagh ne ne ôr nyi?	Tiv offspring oo, you all heard this, and what do you say?
Fulani a bee se oo!	Fulani will eliminate us!
Ôn-Tiv oo! Ne ne ungwa kwagh ne ne ôrnyi?	Tiv offspring oo, you all heard this, and what do you say?
Fulani a bee se oo!	Fulani will eliminate us!
Gomna u Benue oo!	Governor of Benue oo,
We u ungwa kwagh ne u ôr nyi?	you heard this, what have you said?
Fulani a bee se oo!	Fulani will eliminate us!
Mo me pine ne sha zamber,	I'll beseech you all,
ne ne ungwa kwagh ne ne ôrnyi?	you've all heard this; what do you say?
Fulani a bee se oo!	Fulani will eliminate us!
Shi me pine ne sha zamber,	Again I'll beseech you all,
ne ne ungwa kwagh ne ne ôrnyi?	you've all heard this; what do you say?
Fulani a bee se oo!	Fulani will eliminate us!

This song directly calls attention to the conflict situation, challenges inaction and raises alarm of the impending ethnic cleansing. The displaced people first call on the Tiv people generally asking them what they have to say about the conflict situation. In doing that, they call on the Benue State Governor also asking what he has to say about the situation. It is a call and response song wherein the call mentions people and asks the questions meant to sensitize those called and also prick their consciousness to take effective action. The response part articulates the ethnic cleansing agenda and specifically singling out the Fulani as the aggressors.

Song 6

TIV	ENGLISH
Anyôr tar oo! Se saa ve!	It has entered town oo! We are lost!
Agwei nyôr tar oo! Se saa ve!	*Agwei* has entered town oo! We are lost!

Agwei yisa tar ve oo!	*Agwei* has surrounded town oo!
Ortom Agwei yisa tar oo, se saa ve,	Ortom *Agwei* surrounds us, we are lost!
Agwei yisa tar oo se saa ve,	Agwei has entered town oo! We are lost!
Agwei yisa tar ve oo (2x)	Agwei has surrounded town oo!

In this song, the displaced announce the wake of the attacks. They raise an alarm telling the world that the assailants have come and they indeed are lost. "*Ortom*" who is mentioned in line four is the current Governor of Benue State, and the displaced persons consider him as the right person to respond appropriately to their plight. This is not farfetched from the constitutional role of a Governor as the chief security officer of a State. The fact that these alarms are raised to the appropriate authorities and the people still suffer these attacks is another issue entirely about whether constitutional roles and responsibilities are being fulfilled or not, or whether there is a fundamentally inherent problematic with the security framework which makes it difficult for Governors to fulfil this obligation.

4.2.2 Dance and Movement

Dance and creative movement is another genre of cultural performance used by the displaced persons in the study community, Daudu. Whereas dance is rhythmic movement of body within time and space to communicate, movement is not necessarily dance, but a locomotive state wherein the human body fluidly explores its form. Dance requires movement, but movement must not result into dance as the elements of dance may not need to be present before movement is completed. The human body moves and human emotions are moved. Amongst the displaced persons, dance and movement are used simultaneously and they are both steep in improvisation.

Amongst the displaced population, their use of dance involves and expresses emotion, belief, hope and experience through physiological processes; it also provides a means to engage emotions as they emerge through the subtle and often unconscious sensory cues of the body. The creative movements used also communicate their mood which is generally forlorn. The dances are lacking in energy, and projecting a sombre atmosphere which depicts their traumatised states. However, the displaced themselves find positive energy from this energy as they say it helps them release the overwhelming emotions that envelope from their sad memories.

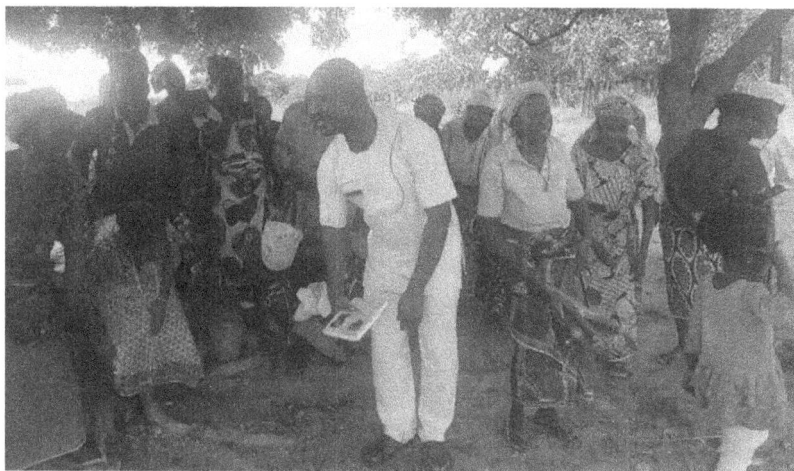

Plate 4: Researcher joined in the slow and sombre dance (Ukuma 2017)

Kwagh u ngu ana ve se mba gberen amo ne kpa shi se vinen yô, shien u genegh ishima ngi a vihi u man we a gberen amo yô, Aôndo ngu A na jijingi u msaaniyol ken a we; nahan shien u ka we a hii u vinen kpa u kera fa ga. Shien u gen je yô, ka u vaan kpashi u vinen. (FGD, St. Francis Mission, Daudu, 14/09/2017)

What makes us sing these songs and dance, sometimes when you are sad and you begin to sing songs, you get enveloped by some soothing feeling, and because of that you do not even know when you begin to dance. Sometimes you will be crying but still dancing. (FGD, *St. Francis Mission, Daudu, 14/09/2017*)

The above excerpt communicates the functional relevance that dancing has on the displaced. The dance is styled after the *Uzagigh* (meaning the very advanced in age), which is a term used to describe the dancing style of old people typically lacking in virility, though graceful. Of course, dance and movement communicating grief and a general sense of disillusionment should be lacking in strength, communicating a weakness that is overwhelming from within the body as is manifest without.

4.2.3 Dramatic Enactments

Dramatic nature of storytelling as practiced in community groups is a prevalent performance mode in Africa. It is usually the narrative content of the storytelling that is approximated into dramatic enactments. Improvised music such as hand-clapping, foot-tapping, vocalizations, or some piece of metal or wood found on the ground. This performance mode is almost innate with the Tiv such that even in the face of turmoil and the traumatizing experiences of the displaced, they find it convenient to dramatize their experiences. What is most interesting here is that the displaced persons did not wait for some professional therapist to prompt them to action or organize them in like manner. From the depths of their emotions, they reached-out to their cultural repertoire and from there adapted existing materials while also creating new ones in order to communicate their situation and also negotiate their well-being.

The dramatic enactments performed by the displaced are completely improvisational. They do not have any structure, just as they are episodic. Anyone from the crowd could start action based on the common experiences they shared as they fled violence. However, no two episodes are played at the same time, once one member of the group starts up an action, the rest of the members join in by doing complimentary action of finding improvised props and other elements to compliment the scene. In this way, several episodes get performed thereby creating an enriching experience of their circumstances.

In the focus group discussion, a participant said all they do is based on what they experienced. According to her:

> When this crisis broke and people started to run, for some of us, not even a cup like this one did we have time to pick. We would just see other people who had run with plenty belongings tied up in a mosquito net. For us we took nothing. We later heard the story of woman whose toddling child fell from her in *Mbagwen* (a sub-clan). She shouted out that the husband should take up the child because she is not stopping for any reason. The husband had asked her earlier to leave but she did not, after a while bullets started flying past through the leaves of trees, that was when in her haste to leave, the baby fell from her hands and she told the husband to take it. That woman abandoned the child and left! That is why even in our drama, it had to be a man who takes the baby after a woman scurries around with it and drops it. No one amongst us creates from imagination. It is based on what have seen and experienced. (FGD, UNHCR Shelter, Daudu, 2018)

What this means is that the displaced persons try to re-enact their lived experiences without exaggeration. Even as spontaneous as their acts are, they are true to their memories and recreate out of the need to share experiences and relief themselves of pent up emotions.

Another interesting scene is where some of the displaced people assume the roles of the assailants in order to heighten the pandemonium being re-enacted. In this scene, one woman begins to shout in Hausa language spoken by the Fulani for ease of communication with other tribes instead of their original Fulfulde. It is impressive that even as they fled, they had the presence of mind to

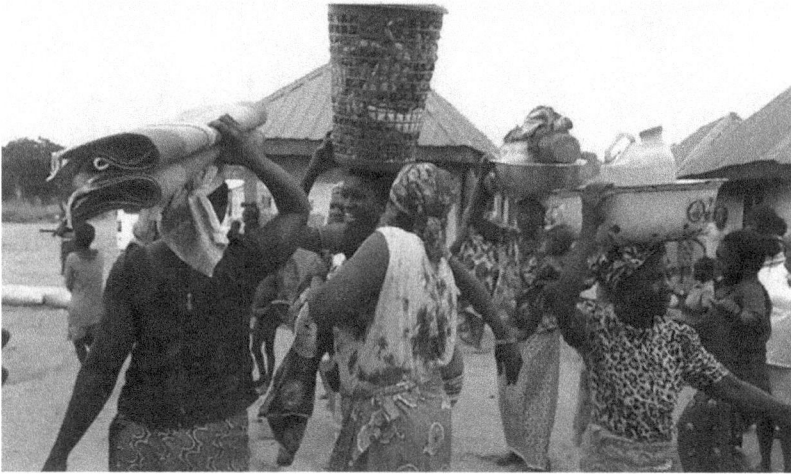

Plate 5: Displaced persons dramatizing how they fled with their belongings (Ukuma 2018, UNHCR Shelter, Daudu)

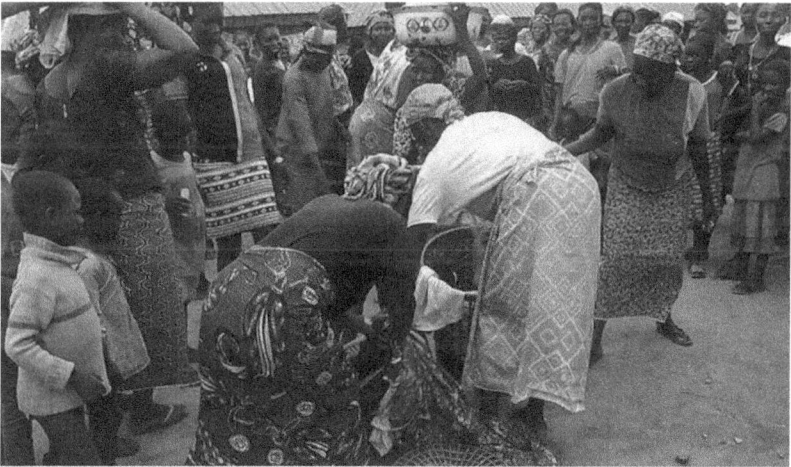

Plate 6: Here, a woman falls with her luggage and another assists her (Ukuma 2018, UNHCR Shelter, Daudu)

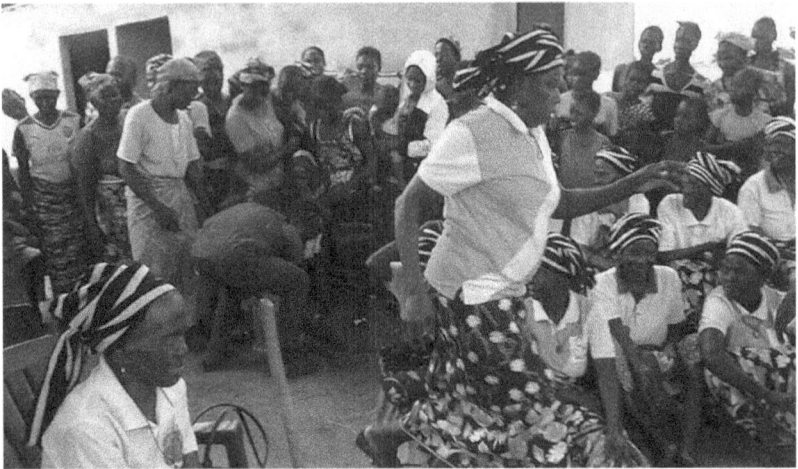

Plate 7: In this scene, the woman in motion is the supposed woman who dropped her baby as she fled. Notice the man in blue behind her picking up the child (Ukuma 2018, UNHCR Shelter, Daudu)

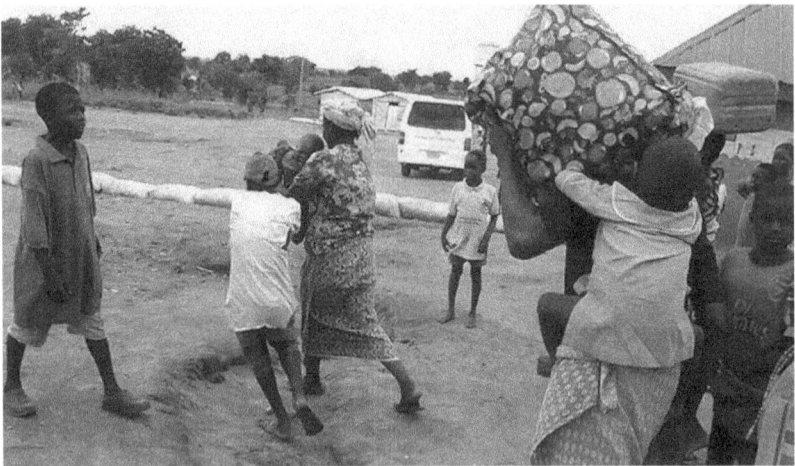

Plate 8: Notice here a man trying to help a woman with her child so she could run faster. Another woman bears the burden of a baby and luggage. All these are spontaneous re-enactments of their experiences (Ukuma 2018, UNHCR Shelter, Daudu)

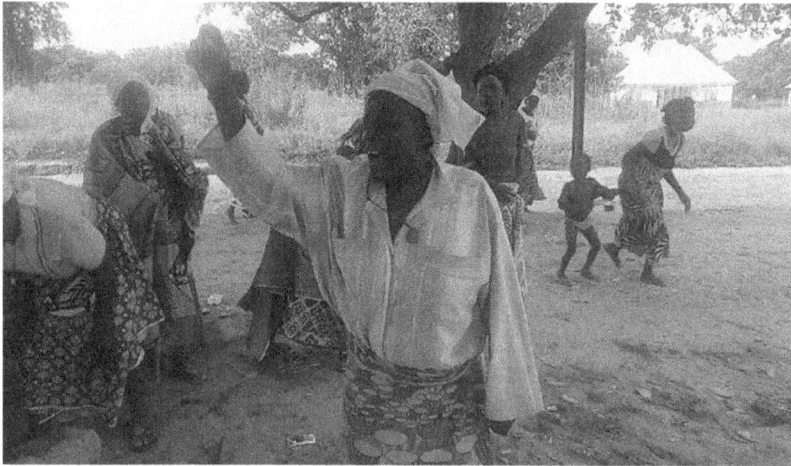

Plate 9: Pictured here is a woman rendering the lines in above excerpt. Notice another woman behind sneaking to safety with a child (Ukuma, St. Francis Mission, Daudu, 14/09/2017)

register what was being said on their heels, it also communicates how very close they came in contact with violence. The woman is heard shouting:

> *Za mu gama de Tibi, Shegye Tibi, za mu kashe su duka; a kama de hanu*
> We will finish the Tiv, useless Tiv, we will kill them all; catch them with your hands...
> (Fieldwork, *St. Francis Mission, Daudu, 14/09/2017*)

This indeed is an example of some of the voices they still hear in their sleep that traumatise them. Such voices bring to mind their close experience with death just as it reminds them of their relations who actually fell to their deaths on account of same voices.

4.3 Contextual Findings

In this section, the findings are presented in relation to the research questions. Thus, the findings relate to how respondents generally describe the role of cultural performances, and the extent of their knowledge on the impact of cultural performances in managing collective trauma. Findings also relate to the application of cultural performances for collective trauma management, the challenges that there is with this application, and approaches to negotiating these challenges. Although findings are structured according to the research questions, references

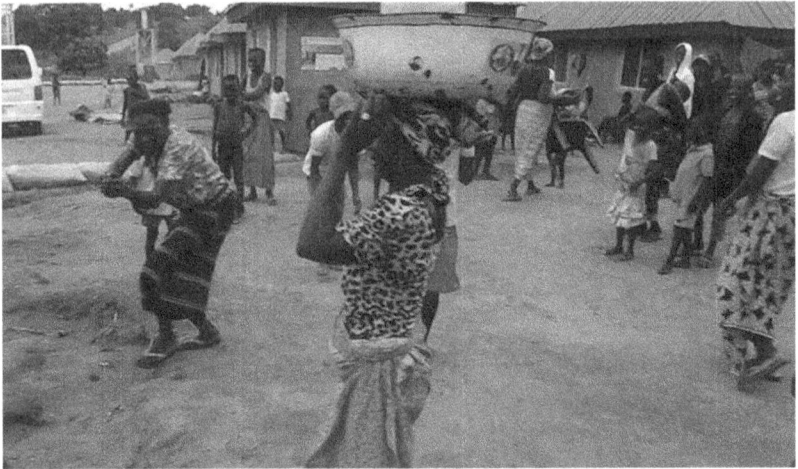

Plate 10: Here the woman on the left bends to take aim at a fleeing resident as the attacker would (Ukuma2018, UNHCR Shelter, Daudu)

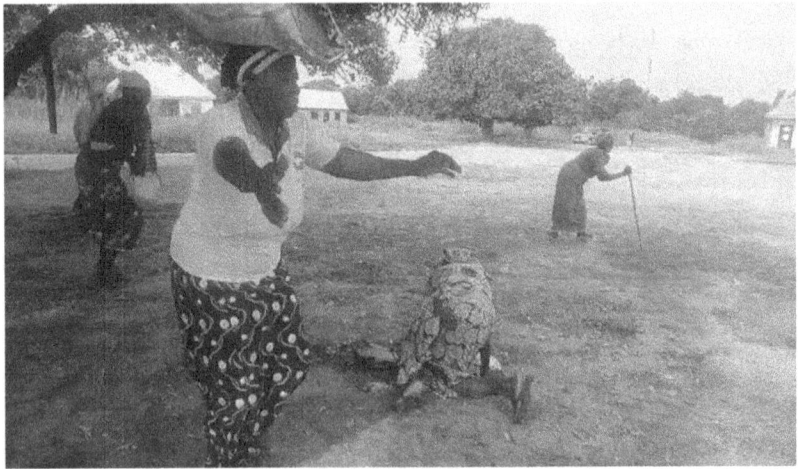

Plate 11: In this scene, a woman falls to the ground as she makes to run, this according to her was what actually happened and she dislocated her ankle in the actual experience. Another woman opens her arms in wait of a child running towards her (Fieldwork, St. Francis Mission, Daudu, 14/09/2017)

are made to data generated from observation where necessary in order to give full understanding of themes.

4.3.1 Functions of Cultural Performances in Daudu Community

The study sought to answer research question one – "What are the functions of cultural performances in Daudu community?". In this regard, a major theme that emanates from the data generated was Identity and this had sub-themes such as propagation, communication, documentation and education.

4.3.1.1 Identity: the issue of identity was central to the respondents in describing the quintessence of cultural performances to them. There was a clear indication by participants in the study that their performances very much represent who they are, whether they are directly saying who they are in the songs and dances, or whether they convey other subtle messages that are peculiar with them or their aspirations, it all sums up to defining who they are. This strong notion of identity was profoundly described by an FGD participant thus: *"well, that is who we are, of course. You can tell from our performances that we are farmers, we are peace loving, we love our brothers, we care about our land. What else?"* This submission resonates with the wider literature on identity construction which point the fact that dance, music, puppetry, masquerading, sculpture, painting and naming are all invaluable in gathering information about peoples or understanding their cultural ideologies (Ezeifeka 2019; Jeannotte 2016; Itulua-Abumere 2014; Ugbem 2013; Cerulo 1997). Participants described the issues of identity in various ways they perceived as crucial.

Propagation was highlighted as a sub-theme of identity. Participants described their performances to be about promoting who they are and projecting this notion to themselves and the world around them. They described the performances as "our thing", "our being", "our practices". A participant was emphatic the "practices mark us out as unique" and "make us easily known". This notion resonated with the participants at the FGD session. This underscores that to the participants, identity is seen to be perceptions or perspectives that are engaged in defining the self, a group or groups, ethnicities, and other social elements that may bind people together. Scholars like Clark (1990), Huntington (1997) and Hult (1999) also hold a similar view as they posit that theoretical constructs emanating from discourse of national identity have been erected around the concept that certain distinct elements mark out a culture and makes the same adaptable to other cultures and that the totality of these elements constitute its national identity.

Another sub-theme for identity was communication. Participants observed that they are able to "tell" or "inform" about their notions of themselves through their performances. In directly "showing" or "demonstrating" elements of their worldview in the performances, or portraying subtle messages or cues embedded in the performances, they "communicate" about who they are, what their worries and fears are, and what their hopes and aspirations are. A respondent noted that "through our singing, we tell that we are farmers". This communication element informs us of the unique characteristics of a given culture's identity, and the extent to which members of such a cultural space identify with, and responds to its unique characteristics.

There was also the issue of documentation. The quintessence of performance being a tool to preserve elements of identity was highlighted. The submission was that these performances record events and happenings within the society, just as they also entrench themselves as the people's way of doing things: of singing, dancing, celebrating, mourning. Participants described this documentation function as being very important vis-à-vis their circumstances as victims of violent conflict. For example, a participant said:

> As we are now, we are disorganized, very many of us cannot write; even those who can do not have that presence of mind to write, because we are a people on the run. So our best option is to record our experiences in songs and dances. This is easy for us and convenient. The songs are easy to learn and we sing them every now and then, so we always remember who we are and what has happened to us (Maakyer2018, UNHCR Shelter, Daudu)

This description is a significant finding in this study because the participants portray a consciousness not just of who they are, but also of what is important to them. The consciousness of what to document and the need to remember are crucial steps in transformative processes.

Education is another function these performances play within the community. In most non-literate settings, knowledge is transmitted through oral forms, lessons are passed from generation to generation using various cultural forms, and these performances are not an exception. They are veritable tools for coding and decoding indigenous knowledge systems. In the case of these displaced persons, the question of memory which is critical to healing and transformation processes is adequately accounted for with these performances.

4.3.2 Extent of Knowledge on the Effect of Cultural Performances in Managing Collective Trauma in Victims of Violent Conflicts

In the attempt to answer question two which sought insights into the extent of knowledge of the effect of cultural performances in managing collective trauma amongst victims of violent conflicts, the study identified varying degrees of knowledge from the different participants. The social workers and academics interviewed demonstrated deep levels of knowledge on the impact of this mechanism and were conscious of its functionality while the victims themselves were equally knowledgeable but it was also a process of discovery for them. Iorapuu (personal communication, 16 March, 2019) asserts that the people themselves, even if they are not saying it, are aware of the effect of cultural performances in managing their traumatic experiences. He posits further that "the people themselves, despite their pains, their traumatic experiences, are able to gather some energy to recall to performances, their pains, trying to console themselves to deal with their shock and their pain, and even encourage themselves that all of this notwithstanding, let's pull together and move on". A social development consultant interviewed asserts that:

> one of the key issues about trauma is that people's sense of options are distorted, or they are struggling to make sense of life, to make sense of living a normal life again, now theatre… has important roles it could play and indeed has played in the past, I remember while growing up, you would attend sometimes the *Kwagh-hir* Festival and you're watching performances that looked so real that it appears that somebody actually experienced a certain thing, or a story is presented, a dramatic presentation gives you an idea of how a certain person overcame a certain situation. Now, what I see such performances do is that one, it provides an environment for entertainment, the very act of entertainment provides an opportunity for emotional release, it gives you an opportunity to move away from the situation of lack of options or distorted options, to a situation where you are able to relax, you're able to be playful, you're able to be playful, you're able to laugh. Psychologically that has very positive effects, but you come out of such an experience more refreshed and better positioned, or better able to think of what the next day should look like. But let's also just imagine that the entertainment presented a story of a very difficult situation that somebody managed to pass through, when that happens the theatrical performance is not only giving you an opportunity to relax and laugh and be refreshed, but it also presents an opportunity of how to deal with the kind of situation you may have passed through. So in a way and this is just starting, but in a way I think yes… cultural performances do have a way of helping to address collective trauma. (N. M. Awuapila personal communication, 21 February, 2018)

The above respondent shares experience as a trained expert in social development, and also relies on his childhood days to give insight into awareness of how cultural performances function in managing trauma. The displaced performers were also emphatic about their awareness of the cultural performance mode. They stated that they would initially pray and wait on God, but they realised that if the Christian songs they sing would offer them succour, then they would try something more encompassing and acceptable by many so that they reach a wider audience. Asked if they have other options to finding succour collectively, a participant said "*ka di msen man amo ne tsô,* meaning, it is just prayer and these song performances.

4.3.3 Applying Cultural Performances in Managing Collective Trauma

This question was about seeing how best cultural performances could function in the management of collective trauma. Responses were sought to elicit the roles of policy, traditional institutions, civil society organizations, and the communities themselves. Different respondents were of different opinions. The role of policy was considered central as it does not only shape government programming but also provides a framework within which other interests can also operate legally. A respondent identified the National Council for Arts and Culture and her sister State Arts Councils, and the National Orientation Agency as lead agencies which should define policy direction in this regard and provide leading implementation action. He reasoned that:

> …the mandate of the Arts Council allows them do whatever they could do to promote all the cultures in the context, and I would say I'd love that they explore much more, they may not have been doing enough… as I see it, as an outsider, there is no conscious drive to promote cultural performances for the purpose we are discussing here today, it is not in the thinking, or the official thinking of these agencies. And the National Orientation Agency is equally a very relevant agency in this regard, but I do not see any evidence that they are thinking of even the national values being integrated in promoting culture for the sake of the topic we are discussing today. (N. M. Awuapila, personal communication, 21 February, 2018)

The issue canvassed here is that agencies might be underperforming or not thinking in line with existential realities that they exist to tackle. The respondent goes ahead to argue that a new agency might be necessary, with a clear policy direction, to harness and harmonise resources and mandates of other relevant agencies in order to drive the mainstreaming of cultural performances in transformative processes, including the management of collective trauma. The respondent submits that:

> imagine if we had an agency for cultural sustainability, such an agency may be working more consciously to support the Arts Council, and collaborate with the National Orientation Agency to develop content that practitioners, experts can then extract and put it to use for the purpose of trauma healing. Unless an agency exist, or an individual, or an organization comes up that makes that their mandate, we may still see people just going their various directions. (N. M. Awuapila, personal communication, 21 February, 2018)

Another respondent agreed with the idea that policy is central to mainstreaming the use of cultural performances in managing trauma. He however differed that consciousness must begin with the traditional institutions first, otherwise mere policy statements will not make any sense. In his opinion,

> Before you talk about the government, there is what the traditional society recognizes, if government creates policy you cannot come and force it on people to do it, it's the traditional rulers recognizing that this is important; it's a way of doing away with our social vices in the state. Yes, this has to start with the villages, in the town let's see how people will start having neighbourhood, let's see how the person next to you, how can you interact with the person, get to understand what the person is going through, the person gets to understand what you are going through... (R. Ibaishwa, personal communication, 26 September, 2018)

On his part, Iorapuu (personal communication, 16 March, 2019) insists that there must be a policy guide which must be taught in schools and also seen in operation in everyday engagements:

> I think there must be a deliberate cultural policy, in the view of experiences that we are having now; one, we need to look at our educational system, its content, what are we teaching our kids, if all along we have been teaching our children borrowed cultures, then we need to come back and deal with what will benefit us directly, so that is one, we need to look at that, a deliberate attempt to do that, and in order to sustain this we must ensure that what we are insisting is thought in schools is what people are practicing in different places, so that there is that consistency, we can't introduce something in schools but do something else differently. In addition to that, we must learn to ensure independence of the traditional institutions, so that they can be held accountable and responsible, so that they too can hold government accountable...

On the role of civil society organizations in application of cultural performances in their work with victims of collective trauma, a respondent opined that:

> Coming to organizations providing psycho-social support, and yes my organization has provided some psycho-social support, but in the IDP camps what I see many organizations do which they call psycho-social support is... more of practices that are brought to us from the outside, so you might have people that organize children to play football,

that organize children to play games, but games that we know are not the kind of games our children growing up in the villages know about, so they do this and it begins and ends with the modules that they have been taught; the conscious attempt to dig into our cultures and bring something that is culturally relevant to enrich the psycho-social support material that they have hasn't been there, but if organizations do a lot of that I'm sure they will come out with content, has my organization done that so far? No, but this interview gives me a reason to say that is an area to investigate more; what do we have culturally that we could use to enrich the psycho-social support we are providing, whether its targeted only to children or to the elderly or to women or to the youths, we need to do more of that than rely on the modules that are brought to us from the outside, and so there is obviously a gap. (N. M. Awuapila, personal communication, 21 February, 2018)

What is crucial in the above excerpt is the recognition that activities so far constituting the psycho-social support work of intervening organizations are replete with practices from foreign contexts. The respondents submit that a conscious attempt must be made to bring out relevant elements from within the cultural contexts to bear on interventions such that the people can conveniently connect to same and are able to retain ample knowledge after intervention programmes round up.

Another important point in this question of application of cultural performances in collective trauma management is that of role of communities experiencing trauma themselves. Respondents recognise that with the experiences of the displaced persons in Daudu, communities in similar circumstances can already get to work. According to Awuapila (personal communication, 21 February, 2018),

where you have a camp and you have people that were already doing this before they met the disaster, they are not going to wait for somebody to tell them because they will know that this has always worked, and by the way, if you are talking about the Tiv people for example, Tiv people in rural communities, including those in towns, I grew up in the town but this was part of our family practice; in the evening, the household will sit together, they tell stories, sometimes it includes dances, they stand up and dance, sometimes the dances are part of a tale that is told, and so the Tiv people value this, they value such entertainment which is seen as part of their lifestyle, so it is possible that where you have people that have lived through these kind of experiences they will do it because they have experienced the benefits of regularly coming together, entertaining themselves, for people like that it's not going to be a distraction, it's going to be a conscious plan to keep themselves entertained, yes.

From the excerpt above it is clear that what needs be done is a clear sensitization agenda that acknowledges the availability and ease of use of cultural performances in collective trauma management contexts. The people themselves seem to be reservoirs of this knowledge system and are predisposed to engaging them for functional purposes.

4.3.4 Challenges of Cultural Performances in Managing Collective Trauma

Perception: one of the issues identified as a challenge to the cultural performance mechanism in managing collective trauma is that of the prevailing perception that art-based approaches are less serious options. Even as these approaches are gaining acceptability globally, the perception still prevails that they are less serious and as such they are given less attention. The general public feeling is that it is pedestrian to ask someone or a group of persons suffering trauma to go and dance or sing. Even from the researcher's experience when sharing about the thrust of his research with random members of the public, this feeling is highlighted. The experience was also that from the host community, it was observed while asking people whether it is important that the displaced persons come together to do dances, to tell their stories, to sing songs, and to create this kind of communal atmosphere, the general response was that of resentment for uthe approach. Even a clinical psychologist who participated in the interviews retorted: "Yes! Even if I am the one, I will certainly feel you are not being serious". He however went ahead to add from a professional view point that awareness must be created and cultivated amongst the people to enable them embrace this approach and open up towards it. Awuapila (personal communication, 21 February, 2018) is also of the opinion that perception is a problem especially

> those who see the cultural performances just as entertainment and so are not taking a lot of thought, serious enough thoughts about how to package the cultural performance to be culturally sensitive but also sensitive to the religious biases of those who should benefit from it.

He Goes further to aver that one could also find some very interesting cultural nuances that challenge such interventions:

> I was speaking with someone and I mentioned that sometimes cultural norms do not permit people to talk openly about certain things, for instance someone might be traumatized by reason of rape, in the face of this violent conflict, but to come and sit and talk about rape is what you cannot find, it's not encouraged in the cultural setup of the people. (N. M. Awuapila, personal communication, 21 February,2018)

The displaced persons themselves are aware that some people think that the cultural performance method is not one to be taken serious. This is first manifested in the adult male population amongst them who think it is a soft approach only fit for women and children. Those who indulge in it however do not care because they feel so strongly about the usefulness of the approach to them.

It therefore follows from the above that the resilience of the traumatised population using the cultural performance mechanism is quintessential in maximising its usefulness.

Structural dynamics: part of the violence suffered by the displaced population is structural. From the perspective of the displaced persons, agents of oppression are present with them and this complicates the challenge with the impact of the cultural performance approach. The police are stationed to guard the camps, but the displaced persons feel they are also there as spies to checkmate them. There is a high level of distrust between the parties. Some of the displaced persons believe that the police, and to some extent the entire security apparatchik of the state, are complicit in the circumstances that have led to their being displaced. As indicated in the conflict overview presented earlier in this work where corruption was pointed out as an enabler of the conflict, the displaced persons feel that the security did not play their part well in averting the unsavoury circumstances they found themselves in. This already puts them on edge with their presence in the camps. Iorapuu (personal communication, 16 March, 2019) opines that:

> …don't forget that the police themselves are part of the structural challenge in the sense that they represent the instrument of oppression. Don't forget also that the people do not even trust the police, and I will like to submit to you that if the people have their way they wouldn't even want the police around them, because where were the police when they were attacked in the first place? …but that also means that in addition to the fear of the police, or the deliberate attempt of the police to disperse them so that they don't get organized, because the instruments of power don't want people to gather together, to speak with one voice, because instruments of power will always remember that numbers mean power from people organized, they are more powerful, they speak with a common voice and they approach issues more collectively. So such a collective gathering is dangerous for them…

Awuapila (personal communication, 21 February, 2018) takes the issue further as he submits that:

> statutory agencies constitute constraints, you mentioned the police and that's true, they tend to be suspicious of any gathering at IDP camps, but it's not only the police, a number of other security agencies and vigilante groups even tend to do a similar thing. But even the agency coordinating humanitarian support sometimes may not be sufficiently informed about the value of this and may see it as… they may make some passing remark about people who want to provide cultural performances as coming to extort money from the IDPs, they see it as an attempt to come and entertain in order to be paid, and so that level of ignorance could also constitute a constraint to people that genuinely

want to come and provide psycho-social support by way of cultural performances, so these things exists.

Another dimension is that the security personnel do not allow them to gather in their numbers as the general perception is that they may be gathering to hatch plans for reprisals or other such things. This obviously challenges the frequency of their using the group performance mode until such a time when the security are preoccupied with something else or some individual or organization visits the camps with donations. The people living in camps therefore have less time to congregate together; it is those who live with relations or friends outside the camps that therefore champion this approach with the creativity involved, they share with those in camps at such opportune times and are also on hand when visitors come. They therefore easily take the lead and the camp dwellers join in, taking a cue from those leading and jumping it with relevant improvisations and blending spontaneity.

Subjectivity: individual dispositions arising from several factors also pose a challenge to the use of cultural performances in the management of collective trauma. Some persons is from the degree of hurt they are nursing, for some it is a belief system while for others is the complexes that come with the perception that the approach is less serious.

From the religious point of view, some persons from the displaced population who identify as devout Christians were not completely averse to the performative mode but would rather sing songs from their Christian denomination. To this, Awuapila (personal communication, 21 February, 2018) says:

> the issue of the respondent that told you "I'm a Christian and I would do this, I would rather sing songs from my denominations", its real. And sometimes when you pay attention to the kind of songs that come from the cultural performances, some of them may be… they may be offensive to certain people, some of the songs are rude, some are raw, and some people that hurts them rather than heal them, and so they may not want to hear that, so those are some of the issues, which again takes us back to the issue of having somebody who mentors these people because now they realize this is not just about entertainment, this is about trauma healing, so if I'm out there to heal the trauma experienced by a collective, for that reason it means I need to be trained sufficiently to go and do a performance that brings people together rather than tears them apart in the course of trying to solve a problem.

Based on the above, it is instructive to note that such a position may be misleading because it is made from sweeping viewpoint and not from the specific context based situation of the displaced persons. From the repertoire of songs, dances and dramatic enactments performed by the displaced persons as collected in the course of fieldwork through audio-visual recordings and undisclosed observation sessions, one can safely submit that there is no profanity or mundane content of some sort in their performances. However, the variegated denominations of Christianity with their prevalent doctrinal prejudices, which to some extent have greatly contributed to the dwindling popularity of cultural performances amongst the Tiv people despite their known usefulness, are directly responsible for blanket profiling of the performances as being profane, fetish and too sacrilegious to be courted or patronised by a "believer".

Subjectivity was also evident in the extent of individual trauma experiences. The gravity of these experiences made some displaced persons shut down completely. This may make such persons withdrawn and never disposed to participating in anything. This cannot mean that the cultural performance mechanism is not effective, but it is rather challenged because the target group may generally suffer this type of severe trauma and may therefore not be disposed to availing themselves for the process.

From the several field visits and performance instances witnessed in the course of this research, it was only on the member check and consensus building day that a certain aged woman came out to participate. Upon inquiry, it was revealed that she had never participated in any activity in the camp, neither did she collect any form of support from anyone, whether material or cash. It was revealed also that she questioned and denounced her faith because even as a widow, in her presence, her remaining family of nine, including her only surviving son with his wife and five children, and two other relations were hacked to death by the marauding herdsmen militia, herself maimed and left for death. The entire camp population was amazed that she would leave from the bathroom straight, soap and sponge in hand, with just her wrapper tied above her breasts to come and join in the ongoing performance. Such was the power of the communal pull the performances had on this profoundly traumatised woman. This is why it is also important to recognise that managing trauma is a process rather than an event, it is not a cure! It will require consistency and persistence for meaningful progress to be made.

4.3.5 Strategies for Effective Use of Cultural Performances in Managing Collective Trauma

This question sought to elicit views on what could be done to enhance the effective use of cultural performances in managing collective trauma. Specific interests were at the levels of government agencies, social structures like family, religion, traditional institutions, the civil society and community members, and the role of researchers.

Responses to the above concerns were concise and direct in that they pointed to the fact that availability of evidence of the potency of this mechanism is what will drive the commitment of other stakeholder groups in promoting and of course mainstreaming the use of cultural performances in transformative processes beyond the pre-set place where they are seen as mere appendages to "more serious" approaches. Awuapila (personal communication, 21 February, 2018) opined that:

> We are in a world where evidence is what people are looking for, and so for cultural performances to rise to the status of being recognized as a contribution to trauma healing, somebody needs to apply evidence, somebody needs to be able to find the evidence that this is really addressing trauma, what kind of trauma? Which level of trauma? Among which target groups?

This means that more efforts needs to be put into researching the efficacy of cultural performances in order to generate adequate evidence that will form the basis for policy reforms, local initiatives and civil society engagements. He explains further that:

> Most of us, if I may say so, have not seen cultural performances as playing key roles in addressing trauma really, they have seen it more from the angle of entertainment and when we see cultural performance as merely entertainment it means we are seeing only a portion of it, I think … maybe not going far enough to talk about policy, but going far enough to say those who are in a position to handle these issues need to make a lot of conscious effort, it's going to require a lot of conscious effort to bring out the fact to those concerned, those who should let cultural performances be applied towards addressing trauma, collective trauma, that this works. This requires some level of expertise, and so until we get to the point of knowing for sure that in this kind of context these are the kind of cultural performances that should go, for this kind of target group these are the kind of cultural performances that should be applied, we need to get to that point. Now what we have is a medley of all kinds of cultural performances presented to people who have not been analyzed in order to say ok these are the people that constitute this group so we have this bit, and this bit, so it fits, we are just throwing it to them and letting them take what they will, and dispose of what they don't…(N. M. Awuapila, personal communication, 21 February, 2018)

The role of research is again highlighted here strongly. The idea is that context must be properly established and culturally sensitive issues isolated through careful research and sifting of offensive material in order to make the mechanism more acceptable and popular with the people. Here, a well-motivated researcher would go into the field clearly with the intention to identify content that can be utilised effectively. Ibaishwa (personal communication, 26 September, 2018) corroborates this line of thinking when he insists that:

> We just take a step back and think about how cultural performances have helped a community here or there, I think, like you said, the resources to apply cultural performances to address trauma are already available in the community. But a lot of the resources are raw and need to be cooked a little bit, so when you have available cultural performances; one is to be able to... sift to identify the ones that are appropriate so the kind of cultural performances that are taken to the people that are displace should only be the ones that are appropriate to their needs, that requires some level of training and expertise to know which one is appropriate.

Here, the question of evidence is reiterated, and the idea of raising consciousness levels highlighted. The community members themselves must be aware of the full impact of cultural performances in times of trauma. This will elicit more supportive dispositions from them and also help the social perception which at present is negative. Awuapila (personal communication, 21 February, 2018) also opined that traditional institutions have a key role to play in that "they could key in... even where there are no opportunities they could actually make these resources known... (and) understood".

Training was another strategic point raised as a way of enhancing the efficacy of cultural performances as a mechanism for collective trauma management. It was opined that relevant government agencies and their agents must be trained strategically such they know understand what it means to work with a traumatised population so they can conduct themselves professionally and also select their cultural materials carefully.

4.4 Findings from Systematic Review of Literature

A pioneer of performance theorist, Goffman, states: "All the world is not, of course, a stage, but the crucial ways in which it isn't are not easy to specify" (1959, p. 72). Of course, on a relative scale, human behaviours occur rarely on a formal stage and constantly on the colloquial level of everyday habits and choices. To better understand how embodied behaviours for a sustainable future currently occur and how they might propagate and evolve, the practices and behaviours of people in their everyday lives must be investigated in a way that values embodied knowledge and the context of behaviour. "Performance-centred research takes as both its subject matter and method the experiencing body situated in time, place, and history" (Conquergood2006, p. 359). Performance theory offers a relational, adaptive lens for analysis of human behaviour that re-centres the human body as the first mode of engagement with the world.

In their discussion of non-representationalist theory (Thrift 1996, 1999b, 1999a, 2000a; Thrift and Dewsbury 2000; see also Nash 2000) Thrift and

Dewsbury (2000) describe the pluralism and open-endedness of life and how those characteristics can be echoed in creative research praxis:

> There is a sense in all of this work of an emphasis on the sense of movement, the kinaesthetic sense, as the way in which we can understand the world and of kinaesthetic space, a fluid space in which no fixed standards of representation exist … Fluids necessarily resist adequate symbolisation and in their movement serve as a constant reminder of the limits of the logic of solids to understand change. Such a conception leads us inevitably to the performing arts, for it is amongst their practices that we find fluid spaces worked up, worked on, and worked out. (Thrift and Dewsbury 2000, p. 19)

A turn to the performing arts as a site of creative embodied praxis also suggests that application of the analytic tools developed around performances is also appropriate in the study of social practices. Similarly to Thrift and Dewsbury's call for the performing arts as a richly dynamic site for social inquiry, and in response to the material 'turn' in social theory, Whatmore describes what she sees as an emerging experimental imperative that creates an "urgent need to supplement the familiar repertoire of humanist methods that rely on generating talk and text with experimental practices that amplify other sensory, bodily, and affective registers and extend the company and modality of what constitutes a research subject" (2006, pp. 606–7). Johnson who argues compellingly that the roots of all meaning are somatic, declares the importance of the arts as a site of meaning-making "where immanent bodily meaning is paramount" (2008, p. 209). He argues that philosophers tend to overlook this rich site of processual engagement because of a bias toward cognitive language processes of meaning creation. But numerous fields in the social sciences and humanities have adopted and adapted the notion of performance in their studies of everyday life, and in fact performance as a topic, metaphor, and as a method has become pervasive in academic studies.

Performance theory has found a home in many diverse fields of study. A co-founder of performance studies, Richard Schechner, embraces the diversity of applications of performance theory and suggests a broadly inclusive definition of performance that "includes[s] play, games, sports, performance in everyday life, and ritual" (1998, p. 357). Another key figure in the establishment of performance studies, Victor Turner, characterized performance as a process of "making, not faking", thus centring performance in a "larger view of culture as constructed, embodied, and processual" (Hamera 2006, p. 46). Therefore we see that performance theory is an apposite pathway to take in the task of making space for embodiment in procedural sustainability work because while performance theory begins in the body, it also embraces plurality, relational meaning, and adaptivity (Schechner 2002, p. 22).

Performance properties are properties inherent to all performances. All performances have an author, whether it is a playwright, an improvising actor, or any model of collaborative authorship in-between the two. The author controls the message of the performance; it is often politically crucial to question who has that power, to ask, "Whose story is it?" (May 2011). And all performances have an audience, though the audience may not be flesh and blood, and may be merely perceived by the performer though not actually extant. The audience could be a recording device or it could be an imagined audience or the performer themselves. All performances are dialogic in that they create a relational bond between a performer and an audience, a correspondence of sorts. And in all performances it is possible to raise the question of authenticity, that is, what are the origins of the performance and its message, and does the performance remain true to its origins or play with the notion of veracity? Of course all of this must occur in a place and time, and the setting of a performance contributes greatly to how the performance is perceived and interpreted. While a setting is most often a physical space, changing technologies are profoundly influencing how we experience a performance in space and time, making it possible for performance to occur at a great distance from the audience. Some performances now only occur in virtual space-time, and the fact remains that the context will always contribute to, and say something about, the qualities and characteristics of the performance itself. The setting also helps indicate to the audience whether the performance is a theatrical construct for the entertainment/educational complex or an everyday performance.

Performance elements are tools and techniques that can be used during a performance to create an effect or outcome. The materials of a performance include elements of the setting (such as set design), physical props, costumes, and light and sound technologies. During a performance, many of these material elements will be taken up as material-semiotic actors that have deep social, personal, or cultural meaning, shaping our practices and attitudes (Haraway 1988). Ritual (or repetition) contains within it many overlapping concepts including rehearsal in a straightforward, theatrical sense, but also ritual as a re-enactment of cultural practices, and repetition in the sense of what Judith Butler calls the performativities of a person in social space (1993, 2004). Humour is a performance element that has great power to engage an audience. Humour is sometimes employed to lighten tense situations or to make difficult tasks (such as truth-telling) more bearable.

In many performances there is an element of play that "articulates the (…) space in which we can act 'as if' and reap its experiential rewards" (Schutzman 2006, p. 290). That is, the performance of an imaginative world can be a learning experience (Huizinga 2004). During a performance, improvisation can occur as a speech act, a movement, material use, or any number of unanticipated but influential alterations. According to Goffman (1959), everyday actions are a continuous series of minute improvisations, and Holland et al state that "improvisations can become the basis for a reformed subjectivity" (2001, p. 18). An archetype is kind of heuristic whereby common personality types or recognizable figures are evident in characters. An archetype performs "the expected" (Hamera 2006, p. 50); we alternately might call this a stereotype. The archetype also contains subversive potential along the lines of Butler's performativities (Butler 2004).

Concepts and Abstractions are less tangible dimensions of our experience upon which performances do work. They can be expressed or internalized by a performer or an audience member, and the effect on concepts and abstractions during or after a performance creates a new context for future performances. At the heart of many performances is the identity of the character, performer, or audience member. Butler's (1993) theory on identity posits that performances of identity can be either transgressive or normative – in either case a story about who we are is being shared. Memory is an "active character" of social performance (Crouch 2003, p. 1956) that is shaped by the inscribing practices of iterative performance on stage and in the everyday. Memory plays a leading role in the processes of cultural continuity, which speaks to the conservation or passing on of lived, embodied knowledge. Cultural continuity is closely linked to ritual and repetition. The spatial dimension of performance physically and culturally frames and defines the meaning of a performance. The relationship of space to place changes over the course of a performance, setting up dynamic relationships between people and places (Tuan 2001). "Space too needs to be thought of as brought into being through performances and as a performative articulation of power" (Gregson and G. Rose 2000, p. 434). Performers are "intrinsically corporeal" and so their performance is dependent on and responsive to the performance site in space-time (Thrift 1996:38). Together, these performance components contribute to the formation and delivery of a message, regardless of whether or not the performance is intentionally political or moral. For example, in eco-dramaturgy, the message is one of "ecological reciprocity and community" (May 2011).

These three categories, "performance properties", "performance elements", and "concepts and abstractions", exist in dynamic and synergistic relationship to one another. Performance elements, added to the inherent Properties of a performance, work on Concepts and Abstractions, in turn creating an altered context for future performances. There is therefore a cycle of influence through which performances with inherent properties become specified by select performance elements, and influence the concepts and abstractions that establish the context for future performances.

Sustainability practices are embedded in, and are produced by, the social and cultural fabric of everyday life and have deep connections (including impacts and motivating variables) to the ecosystem processes that support life. Both the language of performance studies and research approach is intimately compatible with social practice theory that "directs research attention towards the practical accomplishment or 'doing' of everyday practices" (Hargreaves 2011, p. 84) that occur in a complex entanglement of social, cultural, and material elements. Similarly, procedural sustainability that conceives of sustainability as an emergent property resulting from collaborative, deliberative processes clearly defines sustainability as a socially, culturally, and, bodily mediated phenomenon (Robinson 2004, 2008).

Performance is a space of fluid engagement between the things and the people who share it. The displaced persons in Daudu embody this truism in their performance in managing trauma collectively. Their highly spontaneous and improvised skits based on the experiences of violence resonates with Dewsbury's view when he avers that "Performances are venturesome couplings – of carpenter and wood; the companionship of dog and human; the relationship between a crocodile and a bird – that are creative in that they negotiate the new, enabling ways to 'go on'" (2000, p. 493). Note that here Dewsbury is not focused on describing the specific space of theatrical performance, but performance in the Goffman sense that denote the kinds of performances of self-in-the-world we enact everyday (Goffman 1959). Performances on stage and off stage share this sense of mutual becoming, the coupling between performer and space, performer and audience, and of course performer and co-performer.

In all, the songs, dances and dramatic enactments of the displaced persons in Daudu could be seen as a form of performative reflexivity. In Conquergood's terms, performative reflexivity is a condition in which a socio-cultural group, or its most perceptive members acting representatively, turn, bend or reflect back upon themselves, upon the relations, actions, symbols, meanings, codes, roles, statuses, social structures, ethical and legal rules, and other socio-cultural components which make up their public selves (Conquergood2006, p. 360) Indeed, the performances of the displaced in Daudu tell of their relations with the herders, what the herders represent to them, the performances question the passivity of the farmer groups and their sympathizers, just as they comment on the existential threat that is present amongst them.

4.5 Conclusion

This chapter has explored analytically the use of cultural performances as a mechanism for managing collective trauma in the displaced persons in Daudu. The performance forms of music, dance and drama were presented as employed by the displaced persons. Data from focus group discussions, interviews and observations were also presented to the extent of how they support or negate the claim that these performances are useful in managing collective trauma amongst the displaced and fostering community building. It was clear that this mechanism was helpful although challenges of perception, subjectivities and oppressive structures limit the extent of effectiveness.

Findings from literature also indicate that the discourse on creative art therapies is dominated by Western thinking which profiles professionalism in this area without paying attention to non-Western approaches. As such, this mechanism of cultural performances by displaced persons in managing collective trauma at a community level provides insight into other possibilities not reflected in the Western literature.

5 Managing Collective Trauma

This chapter discusses how the idea of managing collective trauma through cultural performances worked out in the context of the displaced persons based on the data presented in the previous chapter. The findings are discussed with a view to connecting the field experience with existing literature.

5.1 Findings

The study found out the following as presented in the sub segments below:

5.1.1 Cultural Performances Help in Managing Collective Trauma

The performances of the displaced persons provide a means for negotiating their well-being by enhancing their healing journey from trauma, promoting inner growth, which goes further to contribute to the creation of a culture of peace.

The bodily-performative practices of the displaced persons relate to real-life events and engaging these practices allows for negotiating topics that may otherwise be impossible to discuss. Both psychotherapeutic and cultural-historical approaches to trauma and creativity aim at either identifying and mourning ruptures in a balanced system, or rectifying those ruptures. This brings to bear the question of empowerment where every member of the group finds authentic voice and finds a way to get across. Creating music draws people together. First there is rhythm which tends to get people in sync. And then from the cultural performance context of the displaced persons, particularly with the songs as earlier presented in the previous chapter, there is always a chorus or refrain of a song which the people know and this enhances heightened participation.

The above position resonates with available literature on the effectiveness of dance and movement therapy as well. Zapata (2015) reports an analysis of the effect of DMT and dance on well-being, mood and affect revealed a small pooled effect size, suggesting that DMT and dance may play a useful role as a contributor to well-being, positive mood, and affect. This is the kind of effect that was studies amongst the displaced persons of Daudu Community in this study. Still, the findings of this study should be interpreted with caution as experiences here were conceived on a general spectrum which included quite different variables such as subjective well-being, affect, mood, and stress.

In previous findings for the effects of dance and DMT on well-being, mood and affect were mostly supportive of DMT and dance. Goodill (2006) and van der Merwe (2010), for example, reported beneficial effects of dance and movement on affect and well-being by reviewing the literature. Their studies attempted to answer the question whether thistype of activity (dance or other) really matter, the obvious answer was a yes, this type of activity seems to matter as seen for example, in the Koch et al. (2007) study using a dance condition, a sports condition (moving up to same level of arousal) and a simulation condition (just listening to the music of the dance); the dance condition improved vitality and decreased depressive affect significantly more than the sports condition and the music listening condition. This study with the displaced persons did not yield different results as it is the improved vitality and decreased depressive affect that give credence to the claim that the performances are potent in managing collective trauma.

5.1.2 Subjective Dispositions Affect Extent of Effect

Amongst the study population in Daudu Community, the men consider the cultural performances of dancing, singing and dramatic enactments as a way of managing collective trauma a less serious mechanism and would rather play cards when they are not engaged with livelihood support activities. This disposition is no doubt rooted in the African masculinities where right from boyhood, the males are socialised to operate within a certain cluster of norms, values and behavioural patterns expressing explicit and implicit expressions of how men should conduct and represent themselves to others. From this kind of background therefore, the men may not only stay away from participating but also retain a bias against the approach which takes root in their subconscious and resists any effect of the cultural performance mechanism that tries to take root from within them.

Religious sentiments inherent in some of the displaced persons determined whether they participated in the cultural performances or not, irrespective of their effect in managing collective trauma. Religious dispositions are crucial especially to devout adherents of Christianity who consider cultural materials to be profane. Even though from the materials encountered in the field, one cannot identify that which is profane, it holds still that cultural performances generally are considered fetish and associated with unbelievers. Therefore, people suffering trauma and who identify as Christians may be averse indulging this approach, except where they find a homogenous group of their kind and they select the material that they deem appropriate according to the dictates of their doctrines.

The individual extent of trauma suffered by different members of the displaced community in Daudu was also of significant importance in understanding the effect of the cultural performances in managing collective trauma amongst them. In as much as trauma is collectively shared, people have suffered varying degrees of hurt and therefore the response to the cultural performance mechanism also varies accordingly.

5.1.3 Communal Lifestyle of Victims Is an Asset

As people who are used to communal life styles, group action helps them respond better to their circumstances as they are able to simulate the communal life styles they are used to. From their communal philosophy, shared burden is considered to be no longer too heavy, so as they continue to group together and perform together and generate positive energies amongst themselves, they feel that not all is lost. This makes dealing with hurtful feeling less severe even if it is momentarily. This resonates directly with Turner's idea of *communitas*.

Communitas which is Latin for "unstructured community" in which people are equal, or the very spirit of community manifests as the cultural performances by the displaced persons of Daudu galvanize an intense community spirit, the feeling of great social equality, solidarity, and togetherness. This indeed typifies a characteristic of people experiencing liminality together.

The positive energies generated by the performances helps them to experience a level of transient humility whereby positions change and people attain different levels of social heights; the usual class differences are broken down through common experiences in a way that makes the "high and mighty" experience what it feels to be "lowly" whereas the "lowly" also comingle freely with the "mighty". This levelling helps in building stronger communities when they emerge from this liminal uncertainty to a new reality. This makes communitas an acute point of community as it takes community to the next level and allows the whole of the community to share a common experience, usually through a rite of passage. This brings everyone onto an equal level, even if you are higher in position, you have been lowered and you know what that is. Turner (1969, p. 132) distinguishes between:

i. *existential or spontaneous communitas*, the transient personal experience of togetherness
ii. *normative communitas*, communitas organized into a permanent social system
iii. *ideological communitas*, which can be applied to many utopian social models

During the liminal stage therefore, normally accepted differences between the participants, such as social class, are often de-emphasized or ignored. A social structure of *communitas* forms: one based on common humanity and equality rather than recognized hierarchy. For example, the circumstances of displacement is a shared experience that is common to the entire population and so social hierarchies collapse, the performances help to foster a communitas that creates the ideal sense of community that hitherto seemed only utopian. In this case of the displaced performers, it is the existential or spontaneous communitas that is at work and could evolve into normative communitas. Village heads are all amongst the displaced population in Daudu, and where they hitherto seems infallible and omnipotent, their present circumstances demystifies them as ordinary human beings who also grieve in pain and loss and could be equally helpless. This levelling experience helps to strengthen the commonalities that bind communities together as against the class differentials that deepen oppressive hierarchies.

5.1.4 Women and Children Are More Open to Using Cultural Performances to Engage Their Trauma

From field interactions, it came up that women and the children are more disposed to the mechanism of cultural performances for managing collective trauma. The men considered it a viable approach but a "less serious one". This can be traced to the cultural socialisation in the communities where men are expected to show strength and be more interested in the very serious affairs of protection and livelihood support. Besides, the Tiv word for doing any of the performative art forms is *"numbe"* and it directly translates as "playing"; the question for those who consider the performances as a less serious approach will therefore be why men should be playing.

5.1.5 Escapism is Crucial

The performances of the displaced persons are a form of escapism from the harsh circumstances that threaten their very existence as human beings and as a group. With specific regards to their destitution and shared sense of loss and victimhood, and beyond the reality that they have been rudely cut off from their "normal" everyday lives due to the conflict situation, the collective psyche of the performing IDPs pushes them to, even if momentarily, indulge in activities that rather engage their thoughts and imaginations in a positive manner. Awuapila (personal communication, 21 February, 2018) opines that:

Go to IDP camps for example, and start a drama presentation, people rush to the occasion, they love to participate, they enjoy all of it and they are not in a hurry to leave.
People are looking for just any opportunity that distracts them from the boring lifestyle they are living in the camps, from the painful experiences that they keep recalling
all through the day. So, that is an indication to me that yes people appreciate cultural
performances.

This is a clear pointer that these cultural performances come in handy to ease of
the burden of hurt and equally bring tangibility to the positively imagined possibilities to their lived experiences.

As a matter of fact, imagination (or fantasy) is an important epistemological
tool that diversifies our vision and perception of reality, as well as reality itself. As
a form of migration and the same way as migration, it carries therapeutic power
and emancipates a person (O'keefe, 2004). The displaced describe their performative experiences as taking their minds of hurt and grief; the performances
help them to forget their pain and anxieties and revel in moments of peace and
aesthetical utopia. This means that the performances simultaneously challenge
and rationalize reality, define its borders, and provide stability into it. The balance created by these performances is essential for the community's healthy
functioning. When neglecting, repressing, and devaluating certain sources of information, such as dreams and myths, one undermines the balance. Repressed
or neglected, as Jung (1992) argued, the messages do not disappear completely,
but "their specific energy disappears into the unconscious with unaccountable
consequences". This suggests that our consciousness merely attempts to evade
the unsavoury contemplation of such happenstance in our lived realities. This is
where these performances provide a platform for the displaced to confront their
realities, acknowledge them and develop positive energies towards negotiating a
new realty for themselves. This resonates with the fact that human beings 'escape'
whether physically or mentally from a place of discomfiture to a place of equa-
nimity, hence the quintessence of fantasy in our world.

5.1.6 Improvisation and Spontaneity as Key Elements

Performative reflexivity describes a process of working through an issue with
the performance-building tools such as narrative, plot, character development,
and denouement or resolution. Through iterative acts and reflexive practice,
"improvisation can become the basis for a reformed subjectivity" (Holland et
al. 2001:18). The cultural performances of the displaced persons in Daudu resonate this thinking. The people suffer collective trauma based on their gruesome encounters with violence. To overcome this situation and reorganize their

lives into meaningful existence, they undertake these performances in a process requiring patience, iteration, and open dialogue. Through these same performances, their ability and willingness to adapt new lifestyles, and methods for deciding upon and enacting change, defining capacity for resilience is tasted and refined. In Grosz's terms, by "enabling the unexpected" (1999, p. 25) to influence our actions on the small scale of everyday activities, the performances of the displaced create for them through improvisation opportunities to refigure social structures and practices (Crouch 2003). Spontaneous as the cultural performances of the displaced are, they are manifestations evolving from performative repertoires, which are embodied practices that are rehearsed, garnered over time from multiple sources, which they now tailor to respond to their particular context of displacement and collective trauma. In this way, their ability to adapt to the world around them is reflected in a series of smaller and larger improvisations that call upon the performative repertoires that open up the "reconfiguring, or reconstitutive, potential of performance" (Crouch 2003, p. 1947). After all, the performative encapsulates the potential to carry forward established and iterated performances into the present moment, and to perform a refiguring, a rupturing of the past through our performance in the present. This occurs through improvisation and adaptation, two fundamental characteristics of learning and development in life, and this does not appear lost on the displaced population as is evident in their performances for collective trauma management.

5.1.7 Community Building in Performance

The displaced persons through their performances are able to foster a strong sense of community amongst themselves. The shared sense of a common problem and a common expressive medium creates a bond that generates positive energies amongst them. Indeed, this cannot be farfetched from the experience people have when they share audience-ship watching a theatre piece together, or a concert, or an art gallery. These shared spaces and experience creates a sense of belonging. Where cues from experiences of others participating in the same event as shared and notes taken of those similar, an instantaneous sense of communality sprouts and waxes stronger as the shared experience endures. Be that as it may, it can be said of the performing IDPs have an even stronger case of communality as participation is heightened on two levels: first they are not mere audiences sharing performance experiences, they are the performance; they create it, consume, and embody it; secondly, they relive their own experiences in these performances thereby creating a more profound atmosphere for bonding.

5.2 A Cultural Performance Model for Managing Collective Trauma

The cultural performance approach of the displaced persons in managing their trauma situation is unique and original to them. It evolved out of the need to respond to an existential reality. The people looked inwards within their cultural repertoire and creative abilities to utilise the performance mode in order to negotiate their collective well-being.

It is instructive to note that creative arts therapies are not popular in Nigeria and are therefore not developed and studied with professionals specialising in them. The approach adopted by these displaced persons is original to them without animation or facilitation by some professional or development agent; it is purely the recognition of the healing properties of performance made manifest in the face of daunting challenges on collective well-being.

From field observation and the group discussions, this researcher observed a rather processual approach to the application of the cultural performance mechanism. It is this process that is described here rather than a prescribed model. Indeed, culture-based approaches should never be prescriptive, and this also resonates with procedural sustainability which articulates a process of defining, learning and adapting to changing conditions and uncertainty. It is in line with this sense of procedural sustainability that this cultural performance model (Fig. 2) for managing collective trauma is proposed. The model is to be interpreted as a process and not as an event with a beginning and end points.

It should be understood that the model is a processual procedure, and it can be applied by humanitarian and development workers, state actors intervening in collective trauma management, and traumatised people who on their own wish to use cultural performances to negotiate their well-being.

At the definition stage, it is crucial to understand the context from the viewpoint of the cultural given of the people, and also the background and dimensions of their hurts which they hope to manage. There may be a plenteous variety of cultural performances but there are certainly those which resonate more with the people, and to ensure maximum participation, it is such performances that should be targeted. The discussion around the context of trauma situation will also create content upon which improvisation and spontaneity will build. This will also help to establish a baseline upon which the impact of the performance mechanism will be measured.

The learning stage is for both the animator and the participants. Here, the central thing is the actual participation. Try-outs should begin with the popular cultural performance forms identified at the definition stage. There should be

		Context: trauma background/dimensions; identify cultural performances that resonate with the people; identify talents that can activate the performances from the group; location, time and mood suitable for tryouts
Define	→	

		Participation: performance with available and disposed persons; highlight of moments that resonate most with the group; allowance for spontaneous co-creation; re-creation; repetition and imaginative contents
Learn	→	

		Interaction: flexibility to suggestions; accommodation of small voices, spontaneity; experience sharing; notes for next loop of participation
Adapt	→	

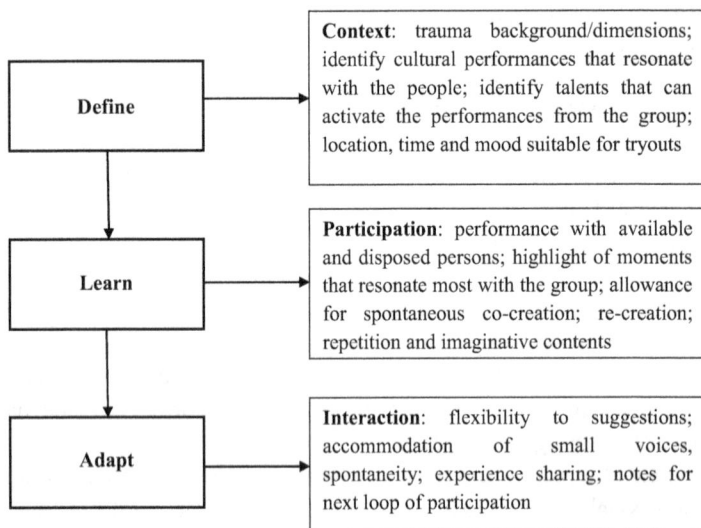

Fig. 2: Ukuma Model for Cultural Performances in Managing Collective Trauma

enough room for spontaneity and improvisation to allow for adequate release of stored up experiences that sustain the trauma. The letting out of steam in such performative atmosphere will generate positive energies, creating new visions and renewing hope in the life ahead. All participants should be able to feel equal so that the process of co-creation will be enhanced; each participant feeling free enough to contribute own experience while ultimately also help own dimension of hurt. With equality in the participation space achieved and spontaneity flowing freely, the performances should be repeated as many times as possible to create ample atmosphere for release of pent up emotions and assimilation of new visions and hopes. It is pertinent to note that the learning stage must be conscious of the elements of recreation and imagination. Members of the group suffering trauma will recreate or reproduce scenarios that reflect their experiences in the circumstances that occasioned their trauma. Such a venture will equally rely critically on the creative imaginations of the members. Through repetition and re-enactment, there will occur an uncommon interaction of passive or subconscious elements with active or conscious thoughts on their lived experiences. Such a robust and performatively unique atmosphere generated through this engaging group activity will cause a profound cathartic effect that will aid psychosocial recovery and well-being.

The next step is adaptation, which should be anchored on interaction. Participants in the process, including animators will have to continue to adapt to the peculiarities of their performative environment. Through interaction, they will know what need to be adjusted, they will be able to check if equality in participation is guaranteed, if spontaneity is being accommodated well enough or whether a particular mode of performance has been overused and should be changed, and so on. This is also the stage where experiences with the exercise are shared and a comparison with the general state of trauma also done. This check will give instant feedback on impact and also inform immensely on next steps. Again, spontaneity is to be highly recognised at this stage such that no one is shut down as this will lead to withdrawal and further trauma.

It should be noted that this model is a process and therefore must not be sequentially followed in the order presented. The various stages identified also loop conveniently into the other and therefore the back and forth cannot be avoided. Anyone using this model must be aware of this. Some of the information that could have come up during the context definition stage may only pop up as a spontaneous input during the performance stage or during the interaction stage as the participants become more comfortable; the same thing may apply during the interaction stage especially if participants become more open due to the positive energies that may have started to build in the group. This is why the understanding that it is a processual activity rather than an event is quintessential to ensuring success.

5.3 The Daudu Experience and Transformation of Farmers/ Herders Conflicts

Transformation of conflict as an approach seeks to create a framework that addresses the content, context and the structure of the relationship. It aspires to create constructive change processes through conflict. Lederach (2003) opines that those processes provide opportunity to learn about patterns and to address relationship structures while providing concrete solutions to presenting issues. He argues further that a transformational approach recognises that conflict is a normal and continuous dynamic within human relationships. Moreover, conflict brings with it potential for constructive change. Although positive change may not happen, and conflict outcomes may result into long-standing cycles or hurts and destruction, the key to transformation is a proactive bias toward seeing conflict as a potential catalyst for growth.

Conflict transformation addressed three levels of differences in need, and these are substantive, procedural and psychological. Since this study is focused on one party (the displaced farmers) in the violent relationship between farmers and herders, the concern here is with the psychological level which reflects how parties feel about issues, and may involve values, relationships, emotions, behaviour and personalities.

The psychological issues of interest here are the personal and emotional aspects. This underscores mind-set issues that require a resetting of the mind to become more predisposed towards other transformational activities like mediation. In the Daudu context, one finds a mass of displaced persons with various degrees of hurt. It therefore follows that this hurting population must attain a certain level of emotional stability before other transformational activities or even resolution efforts will make sense to them. So far, the self-help mode of using cultural performances to mitigate their trauma is considered here as a positive thing that has a long time effect on the possible resolution on the conflict in the future.

Within the creative space where these displaced persons perform, they are able to reflect on the causes and actors within the conflict spectrum and appreciate better the situation. The performances also help them to ease off and release the horrible experiences they have bottled up, as well as the charged up anger simmers within them towards the perceived enemy. The moments of momentary power as they take charge of their lives and decide things within the creative space offers a glimpse of hope in places where it was once only darkness, some voice where it was only silence.

The release of these emotions is quite important to the transformation of this conflict in that it is when these feelings of bitterness, the pains of loss and the disorientation of displacement are eased out of the human body that the ideals of tranquillity, harmony and reconciliation can find entry into a person.

5.4 The Cultural Sustainability and Community Building Implication

A fundamental truth that undergirds the submissions here about the relationship of cultural sustainability and cultural performances in managing collective trauma is that human behaviour and activities are culturally embedded. What this means is that the lifestyles and livelihood activities of the farmers and herders are all rooted in a cultural practices. The cultural performances mechanism of the displaced farmers in managing their collective trauma is equally embedded in culture. It therefore follows that culture is a currency and/or necessity for the rest of sustainability discourse.

On the other hand, conflicts destroy both tangible and intangible heritage. Cultural practices are abandoned and/or forgotten as things are either physically destroyed or people have no time and space to continue there "normal" cultural practices, and without practice, intangible aspects of culture particularly are wont to go extinct.

Culture is therefore not only central to the transformation of the conflict, but also crucial in further development plans. The performances equally connect to the principles of culturally sustainable development as outlined by Throsby (2017). This reflects in three of the five principles as follows:

i. Intergenerational Equity: this is about guaranteeing future availability of cultural forms, both tangible and intangible. There can be no better way of exemplifying this, than a people in the middle of a conflict situation finding relevance for their cultural performance forms and engaging them functionally even to address their immediate challenges of emotional well-being. This will not only ensure that the forms do not go extinct, but also put the forms to task to carry along with them the events of the time into the future.

ii. Intra-generational Equity: this underscores the importance of cultural production and consumption being available to everyone without discriminations. To this end, the performances of the displaced persons are communal and inclusive. They are open performances by the people and for them; a free for all that enlists without restriction as long as members find participating in them to be relevant to them. They performance are open to all without any segregations of sex, class, caste, abilities, and so on.

iii. Importance of Diversity: this is about ensuring that there is space for cultural diversity in all forms. The performances of the displaced persons contribute to diversity subject as they project their identity and contribute to the diversity pool. At the same time, these performances also draw attention to other in the conflict context. No doubt, the performances are about the displaced and the circumstances around their displacement. This means that mention is made of the other party in the conflict even though their identity may not be have been robustly projected. However, this again draws attention to the fact that there is another and this too adds to the diversity subject.

Furthermore, it is the considered opinion of this researcher that cultural performances are quintessential to the future of sustainability studies and praxis. It is highly unlikely that sustainability will be achieved through top-down initiatives and the provision of expert-derived information. There is, of course, a role for information and a need for experts to study the science of climate change and the anthropogenic impacts of our actions, however, a definition of the sustainable future equally requires the inclusion of cultural worldviews, social norms and values. Sustainability emerges where experts and non-experts come together to collectively explore the values, societal beliefs, scientific facts, and governance options that describe the sustainable future. In this model the role of the expert is decentred from being the source of authoritative knowledge conveyed to the audience, and in its place the processes and outcomes of collective conversation gain significance. This is the difference between substantive sustainability, that describes the global-scale achievement of balancing ecological, economic, social, and cultural imperatives, and procedural sustainability that seeks sustainability in the social practices of people, groups, and institutions on the ground (Robinson 2004; Robinson and Tansey 2006).

Matter-of-factly, the strategy to authoritatively state what practices and choices are necessary for sustainability (the information-provision model) has not produced transformative change of the magnitude necessary to satisfy substantive imperatives (Owens 2000; Owens and Driffill 2008), therefore we must explore an alternative framing of sustainability that can more powerfully integrate the concerns and desires of people whose practices will build toward a sustainable or unsustainable future.

Another point to consider is the thinking-space that cultural performance avails. Thinking-space is an embodied act of performing relationships in space that embraces possibility and fluidity. It is process oriented rather than ends oriented, and the outcome is a different valuation of embodied action than as a mere means to an end. In performance theory we also find this distinction between the lived moment of thinking-space and the document or record produced by thinking about space:

> Performance's only life is in the present. Performance cannot be saved, recorded, documented, or otherwise participate in the circulation of representations of representations: once it does so, it becomes something other than performance. To the degree that performance attempts to enter the economy of reproduction it betrays and lessens the promise of its own ontology. Performance's being, like the ontology of subjectivity, (…) becomes itself through disappearance. (Phelan 1993, p. 146)

This concept, or rather, this praxis, thinking-space, clearly resonates with the claim by Thrift and Dewsbury that by turning to the embodied, kinaesthetic moment as the moment of production (rather than abstract theorization after the kinaesthetic moment), "leads us inevitably to the performing arts, for it is amongst their practices that we find fluid spaces worked up, worked on, and worked out" (Thrift and Dewsbury 2000, p. 19). But isn't the act of performance, in the sense of the performing arts such as dance, theatre, and live music, simply the act of doing art? And by this I mean to ask, is it in the creative moment of aesthetic performance that space for reflection and emergent dialogue is produced? If this is so, then performances outside of the performing arts offer the same potential for creatively thinking-space in the kinaesthetic moment.

If the life of a performance is fleeting and ephemeral, as Phelan says, "performance's only life is in the present" (1993, p. 146), then the researcher is faced with a temporal conundrum: every performance, even a reiteration of a previous performance, exists solely in the moment and very few traces of the performance are retained in documents or records. What, then, exists as 'data' for researchers to take up, except perhaps memory. "Through repeated exposure to situations, places, objects, etc. we commit to memory the sensations, emotions and practices that these elicit in the body, whether we are conscious of this or not" (Merchant 2011, p. 63). In this way we build and carry experiential memories with us at all times that "operate as an active character of performativity" (Crouch 2003, p. 1956). The power of embodied memory makes us capable of 'knowing' things in a bodily way even when our engagement is only partial (Merchant 2011), for example, although engagement with a photograph is only partial because it directly engages only our visual organs, seeing the image can call up other sensory stimulations and socio-cultural and spatial contexts not visibly present in the image. Further, viewing images of your own experiences provides "an extension of embodied existence (…) by means of a (albeit compromised) re-living and differently situated (…) view of a previous engagement with the world" (Merchant 2011, p. 64). Photographic documentation of the event cannot possibly preserve the lived experience of the collaborative, dialogic work accomplished during a performance but Martin claims that a practice of documentation can potentially "recognise the disruptive effects of the work of participation lost to representation" (1997, p. 321).

It is not out of place to agree with Thrift (2000) that watching recordings of a performance or reading the resulting document not only alters the performance but establishes a different aesthetic of performance, but at the same time one may extend this line of argument to add that the traces of a performance, such as photographic images, new and different though their aesthetic may be, can be interpreted up against the experiential memory of the original performance to potentially expose new insights.

5.5 The Cultural Policy Imperative

From the findings in the study, it was clear that cultural policy is a veritable tool to drive the connection between cultural performance and collective trauma management, and indeed with all forms of societal transformation. It was clear from responses there are no clear policies giving directions even to agencies of government that could take up such responsibilities directly, or at least sensitize the general population to do so. This resonates with the position of Schneider (2014, p. 18) that the importance of art and culture for the individual and the state can only be fully appreciated when there are in place culture policies that give a particular "boost to cultural participation".

Although Iorapuu (personal communication, 16 March, 2019) recognised that challenge with a policy targeting unpredictable occurrences when he says "people don't sit and deliberately plan that, okay, let's have a cultural policy on insecurity, that we hope that we will be attacked one day so let's begin to do that", he goes on to submit thus:

> I think there must be a deliberate cultural policy, in the view of experiences that we are having now; one, we need to look at our educational system, its content, what are we teaching our kids, if all along we have been teaching our children borrowed cultures, then we need to come back and deal with what will benefit us directly... we need to look at that, a deliberate attempt to do that, and in order to sustain this we must ensure that what we are insisting is thought in schools is what people are practicing in different places, so that there is that consistency, we can't introduce something in schools but do something else differently. In addition to that, we must learn to ensure independence of the traditional institutions, so that they can be held accountable and responsible, so that they too can hold government accountable...

So the issue of cultural policy is necessary, and talking about cultural policy, it's not to be said to mean a policy that will disenfranchise people, but a policy that will ensure respect for one another, a policy that will ensure respect for the other, ... and the other here could mean whether you are gay, whether you are lesbian and so on and so forth ... above all, a policy that will make us recognize that we are human beings, and I think this one of the greatest mistakes in this country today, the lack of respect for different cultures, it's a fundamental thing.

This again point to the inadequacies of Nigeria's cultural policy document as it lacks the potency for the coordination and control of complex social systems and the organisation of cultural diversity and cultural participation. Even though "not everyone is able and willing to draw reassurance from artistic expressions" (Schneider 2014, p. 19), it is crucial that the enabling frameworks are available in their most helpfully operation state such that those who find them useful could maximise gains from them.

In the sustainable development parlance, the implications of cultural rights cannot also be overlooked in the framing of cultural policies. Delgado (2001) reasons that cultural rights have in some contexts come to replace or complement other cultural policy rationales, including those concerned with the economic and social impacts of culture. This underscores why the cultural rights of the Daudu Community people also need to be protected and guaranteed under a new Nigerian cultural policy that mainstreams culture in transformation processes. For such a cultural policy that considers the serious question of cultural rights from a perspective concerned with sustainable development and cultural sustainability, Portolés and Šešić (2017) present five areas for action which include:

i. Access to and participation in cultural activities
ii. Participation in policy decision-making and management
iii. Addressing the obstacles that prevent participation in cultural life
iv. Protection of minorities and threatened identities and expressions, and
v. Protection of cultural resources, rights, and activities which may be put at risk by policies in other areas.

For the Daudu Community studies in this research, the concern with addressing obstacles that prevent participation in cultural life resonates more, in that the displaced persons are cut off from their cultural space and even where they attempt to express themselves through cultural performance as a way of mitigating their trauma, they are confronted with structural challenges like the police suspecting them to be planning reprisals. In a precarious situation, it cultural life which include identities and expressions become threatened and need protection through the instrument of a cultural policy action that is tailored to achieve sustainable development and cultural sustainability.

In view of the foregoing, it is clear that culture and the arts can only fulfil its role in enhancing transformational processes only when they are situated within the framing of international protocols and declarations, until such a time (and it should be urgent) when Nigeria's cultural policy document is reviewed to reflect present realities and the global outlook of culture as a facilitator and enabler of development.

5.6 Conclusion

This chapter discussed the findings of the research and tried to connect same with existing literature. The implication of these findings on cultural sustainability and community building are also discussed as well as the impact of the cultural performance mechanism on the transformation of the farmers/herders conflicts. Discussions in this chapter have prepared grounds for conclusions to be drawn about the research in the next chapter.

6 Cultural Performances, Collective Trauma Management, Cultural Sustainability and Policy: Conclusion and Outlook

This chapter presents a summary of the research after which a conclusion is drawn. The limitations of the study are also presented alongside contribution to knowledge and suggestions for further research. After that recommendations are given.

6.1 Summary

This research explored the phenomenon of cultural performances with a view to establishing their effect on the collective trauma experienced amongst displaced persons as found in the Daudu Community of Benue State. The research problem was defined around the dearth of scientific studies in Africa interrogating the use of art-based approaches in conflict transformation and especially in managing collective trauma arising from these conflicts, particularly in Nigeria. The arguments that the creative representation and aestheticisation of trauma and the reception of such creative works are very complex, in particular when considering representations of African trauma and conflict created outside the continent, through global news networks, popular media and cultural industries were relied upon to deepen the need for a holistically African contextual research on cultural forms and trauma from conflicts on the continent. The argument goes further that "many representations of African conflict by non-Africans, for example mainstream Hollywood films using African atrocities as a backdrop, have not been useful in creating a multifaceted view of the continent. Rather they have led to the desensitization of viewers, promoting voyeurism and a type of 'atrocity tourism', both real... and imagined..." (Bisschoff and Van de Peer (2017, p. 5). Similarly, there is the fact that ethnomusicology has not adequately lent itself to healthcare-oriented research, just as creative arts therapies have also been dominated by Western forms and practices. Put these required attention from a non-Western research context in order to attempt to bridge the gap. The other concern was also to investigate the effect of cultural performances on conflict transformation with a view to promoting this authentically African bottom-up approach to negotiating collective trauma.

The research endeavour sought answers to questions bothering on the role of cultural performances in the Daudu Community, the extent of awareness on cultural performances as a tool for managing collective trauma, the application of cultural performances in managing collective trauma and the challenges that come with it, strategies for mitigating these challenges including the role of cultural policy in this.

Literature survey explored the concepts that are crucial to understanding the background and disciplinary location of the research. This also helped to establish the gaps mentioned in the statement of the research problem, and what the current research will do to contribute towards filling them. Perspectives on cultural performances, cultural sustainability, community building, collective trauma and collective healing, performative therapy were explored, and a spatio-temporal exploration of the conflict between farmers and herders also provided.

Performance theory and social practice theory were used to anchor the analysis and discussions in the study. With performance theory, the strands of liminality and reflexivity were found crucial in exploring the state of uncertainty that the traumatised population found themselves in, and the interface that their performances provide for them to see themselves and recognise challenges and changes that should occur within their body politic. The social practice theory helped to foreground cultural performance as a key element in sustainability discourse.

With the descriptive ethnography approach adopted, through the instruments of interviews, focus group descriptions, observations and performance ethnography, the study found from its analysis that cultural performances are quite helpful in managing collective trauma and fostering sustainable community building. It was also a finding that subjectivities such as religion, gender, and extent of trauma suffered all impact the extent of impact the mechanism has on victims. The role of research in generating more evidence on the efficacy of this approach so as to provide adequate ground for advocacy on mainstreaming it in the programmes of government and civil society organization was identified as a key strategy for mitigating the challenges that come with utilising this approach.

In view of the above, the study suggests that further research be done in several other cultural contexts, including multicultural contexts in order to generate and deepen the evidence of the effectiveness of this mechanism. The conclusion on the study is discussed in the next segment.

6.2 Conclusion

The thrust of this study is the generation of evidence on the effect of non-Western approach to well-being as seen in the role cultural performances have played in managing collective trauma amongst displaced persons in Daudu Community of Benue State. The evidence further underscores the notion that bottom-up approaches that are context specific best suit any sustainable development initiative as transplanting of context through predesigned templates can be problematic and does not empower the target population.

One of the major contributions of this research is the novel assembly and integration of literatures in order to begin to flesh out how sustainability is embodied and performed from an African cultural context. This study has shown here that the worldview embraced by, and common to, the concepts introduced here including sustainability as an emergent property, social practice theory, the embodiment paradigm, and performance theory, is defined by its acceptance of multiple partial knowledge and the essential need to connect theory with lived reality. This resonates with the position that "rather than aiming to produce sustainable citizens,… it is perhaps the making of sustainable performances which should take centre stage" (Horton 2003, p. 75).

To denote the actual, physical actions of a practice, social practice theory uses the term performance. A performance is the actual enactment of a practice by a 'carrier' of the practice (Hargreaves 2011; Warde 2004, 2005). For example, one who is a carrier of the social practice masquerade displays, while performing a particular masquerade, calls upon his knowledge masquerade movement including the cues and codes developed overtime for such a masquerade. The performer's embodied skills of manipulating the masquerade paraphernalia and staying dexterous even while performing a complex routine, the discipline to stay in character even when experiencing a certain discomfort until there is an opportune time, plus his ability to gauge the social requirements of engaging and interacting with the participating audience as well as his performing party, who in their own way are also performing the masquerade practice all sums up as one masquerade experience that fits the description of social practice. This example demonstrates Schatzki's definition of practices as "embodied, materially mediated arrays, and shared meanings" (2001, p. 3). In social practice theory, the embodied dimension of life has intrinsic value and it is through embodied performances of social practices that transformative change can occur because "when practices change they do so as an emergent outcome of the actions and inactions of all (including materials and infrastructures, not only humans) involved" (Shove and Walker 2010, p. 475). Although social practices are collective, widespread, and emergent across large spatial and temporal scales, the carriers of practice are not completely submissive to their forces and can influence the form and direction of practices with agentic intention. Hargreaves explains, "despite their considerable inertia, change in practices emerges both from the inside – as practitioners contest and resist routines and conventions and as they improvise new doings and sayings in new situations – and also from the outside, as different practices come into contact with each other" (2011, p. 83). Social practice theory offers a lot of potential as a useful way to think about and research how sustainability is embodied and performed.

From the foregoing therefore, conceiving of sustainability behaviours as embodied social practices creates possibilities for new perspectives on the processes of social change, on temporal and spatial relationships that inform and are produced by practices, and on our embodied connection to the material, social and cultural dimensions of the sustainable future, the iterative potential of performance can potentially subvert current practices of unsustainability; and this could be both in terms of the performance of everyday activities, and in terms of how a performative act – done with intention for an audience – can be a transformative intervention. The performances of everyday life are "artful as well as taken-for-granted," (Thrift 1996, p. 18). And, in their routine iteration, everyday actions that exist in the fabric of social practices contain the power to subvert, in that, performativities contain the possibility of being done differently (Butler 1990; Cream 1995; Gregson and G. Rose 2000).

6.3 Contribution to Knowledge

This research investigated the effect of cultural performances on managing collective trauma amongst displaced persons. It explored a bottom-up initiative of a displaced people where they employed the expressive arts of dance, music and drama from their cultural contexts in order to negotiate for themselves their well-being. This research endeavour has contributed to the body of knowledge in the following way:

> Evidence on the effect of cultural performance on managing collective trauma was generated. The experiences of the traumatised population studied are documented and described from their cultural perspective. This enabled the researcher to propose a model with which similar phenomena could be explored in others contexts.

The study also generated evidence on cultural performance as a tool for conflict transformation. The transformation of conflicts is a process that is profoundly connected with the personal and emotional aspects of the disputants.

With this study, there is evidence that the transformation process can actually begin with one party in the dispute. When personnel peace and emotional stability is achieved on the one side with bottled up angst and charged emotions are released through engaging performative process, individuals or groups becomes more disposed to meeting with each other to and allow for further transformation processes to be carried through from a less combative standpoint.

The study also proposed a model for using cultural performance in managing collective trauma. This contribution is considered novel in that it provides a framework of operation for those who are not even conversant with a particular cultural context where they have to work. The model is simple and based on procedural sustainability thinking which is processual.

The study also provided evidence on the creative arts practices that exist in Africa, the research recognises them as "performative therapy". The context is uniquely African and is different from the creative arts therapies practiced in Europe and America where professionals take on clients work through a recovery process to the desired state. This is highly standardised and studied with degrees awarded. The performative therapy is communal and available to everyone and can be used by everyone. Its techniques are simple and are intrinsic in the cultural life of the people. Even where individuals such as "traditional doctors" or "medicine men" or "priests" appropriate to themselves such powers to "heal", it is the community that validates or nullifies such a claim.

The study has also contributed to literature on a number of levels. Literature on cultural performance and trauma from an African perspective has been generated; this includes particularly literature on cultural performance and collective trauma management. The highlight is on the community-based approach where a group of people suffering trauma of the same kind pull themselves together and initiate a performative process that is quintessential to their journey towards recovery. The evidence from the research shows this approach as effective and can only be explored further.

There is also literature on cultural sustainability from an African context. Discourses on cultural sustainability are not much in Nigeria at least. This study has generated literature on the subject and equally demonstrated the potential of cultural performances to provide both the material for the discourse, and the outlet for culturally sustainable practices.

Another contribution is the evidence on cultural performance as a veritable tool for community building. Displaced as the study population was, cultural performances helped them to forge a profound sense of community and also enabled them to experience what Turner (1967) calls "existential communitas".

With such an experience, it can only be hoped that it will leave with them enduring tenets that will foster sustainable community building.

The study also established grounds for policy advocacy. Beyond the known fact that Nigeria's cultural policy is an old document which is overdue for review; the study establishes a case of a certain crucial area that must not be left out in the review process. This is in the area of mainstreaming cultural performances in line with the sustainable development thinking.

6.4 Limitations of Study

The time-bound nature of a degree awarding research does not always give enough room for the prolonged observation or extended investigation of a phenomenon. This was also the case with this research. Therefore, the effect of cultural performance on the collective trauma of the people in the long term could not be determined. Findings as presented here are based on the moments of engagement with the study population. However, the study recognises that human behaviour is dynamic and several factors combine to influence this at different times.

The study also considers it a limitation that one case study was used. Multiple cases would have helped to make a stronger case for the mainstreaming of cultural performances in sustainability discourses and practices across transformation processes within Africa.

Another limitation is seen in the non-disaggregation of the study population. An approach aggregating the study population according to gender, age and other dimensions would have brought out a more profound perspective based on the different experiences of these categorizations.

6.5 Suggestions for Further Research

From the findings of this research and the challenges that arose in its course, it is important that further research is made, and here, three areas are suggested.

Firstly, more research needs to be made into this phenomenon of cultural performances and the management of collective trauma especially with the proposed model to generate more evidence on its effect. With more evidence of the effect of the cultural performances model established, even quantitative approaches could be employed to determine numbers with which generalizations could be made or otherwise.

Secondly, it is suggested that research amongst the herder communities too should be done to establish the presence and usefulness or otherwise of the cultural performance phenomenon in managing collective trauma or other conflict transformation concerns amongst them. This will further unveil dimensions to the conflict which are rooted in culture and equally provide useful information that will be handy in any initiative that targets the transformation of the conflict between farmers and herders.

Thirdly, the cultural performance mechanism in managing collective trauma should be further examined in aggregated populations to elicit more in-depth perspectives. Certainly, the experiences of children, youth, women, men, aged and other categorizations cannot be the same even if they face the same challenge. Insights into this can only be gotten when the population is aggregated and studied in such independent units.

6.6 Recommendations

This study recommends the following:

i. The civil society, community leaders and government should pay deliberate attention to cultural performances as a mechanism for managing collective trauma, as well as in transformation processes and community building;

ii. Civil society organizations intervening in conflict areas, especially in providing psycho-social support should look utilising cultural material available within the contextual space instead of the present mode of transplanting templates from other contexts which most times do not resonate well with the people and impact is therefore superficial. A culture-based approach will not only address the problem from a familiar context, but will also leave the people more empowered as they would not be left grappling to imbibe and utilise materials form contexts other than theirs;

iii. Researchers must do more to generate evidence that support the use of cultural materials in line with sustainable development thinking. Such evidence must include experiments with models in order to demonstrate their practicability, successes and challenges so as to inform advocacy and policy direction;

iv. Community leaders must put premium value on cultural performance approaches in negotiating challenging issues like collective trauma management, so as to encourage their constant engagement and subsequent positive perception about them;

v. Advocacy to policy makers and implementers, and sensitization across the communities should be embarked upon by activists and civil society organizations so as to create awareness about the impact of the cultural performance mode in collective trauma management, conflict transformation and other sustainable development concerns so as to mainstream, deepen and popularise the approach.

References

Agande, B. (2017, April 20). Army Launches Operation Harbin Kunama II in Southern Kaduna. *Vanguard News*. Retrieved from https://www.vanguardngr.com/2017/04/army-launches-operation-harbin-kunama-ii-southern-kaduna/

Akerele, C. (2011). "Of national policy on cultural development". *Nigerian Tribune*. April 11.

Amankulor, J. N. (1985). "Festival theatre in traditional African society: An Igbo case study". In Ihekweazu, E. (Ed.) *Readings in African humanities, traditional and modern culture*. Enugu, Nigeria: Fourth Dimension.

Amit, V. (Ed.) (2002). *Realizing community: Concepts, social relationships and sentiments*. London: Routledge. An Ordinary Day (2007), (Unpublished).

Anyanwu, C. (2019). "Nigeria's cultural policy and the needs of the performing arts". *International Review of Humanities Studies,4* (2): 717–727.

Arvanitakis, J. (2008). "Staging Maralinga and looking for community (or why we must desire community before we can find it)". *Research in Drama Education: The Journal of Applied Theatre and Performance*, 13 (3): 295–306.

Bagu, C. and Smith, K. (2017). *Past is prologue: Criminality and reprisal attacks in the middle belt of Nigeria*. Nigeria: Search for Common Ground.

Bauer, J. M. (2013). "Theatre and community: Healing functions of theatre in society". Diss. University of Missouri.

Bauman, Z. (2001). *Community: Seeking safety in an insecure world*. Cambridge: Polity Press.

Bauman, Z. (2004). *Wasted lives: Modernity and its outcasts*. Cambridge: Polity Press.

Becker, H. (1963). *Outsiders: Studies in the Sociology of Deviance*. New York: Free Press, 64 (2).

Bernard, P., Charafeddine, R., Frohlich, K. L., Daniel, M. Kestens, Y., Potvin, L.. (2007). "Health inequalities and place: A theoretical conception of neighbourhood". *Social Science and Medicine*, 65(9): 1839–1852.

Benue State Emergency Management Agency (2018). "Update on Farmer-Herder Conflicts in Benue State, June". Unpublished report.

Bisschoff, L. and Van der Peer, S. (Eds.) (2017). *Art and trauma in Africa: Representations of reconciliation in music, visual arts, literature and film*. Series: International library of cultural studies. I.B. Tauris: London.

Blackman, L. and Venn, C. (2010). "Affect". *Body & Society*, 16(1):7–28. Retrieved May 3, 2012.

Blackman, S. (2004). *Chilling out: The cultural politics of substance consumption, youth and drug policy.* Maidenhead/New York: McGrawHill-Open University Press.

Blake, J. (1999). "Overcoming the 'value-action gap' in environmental policy: Tensions between national policy and local experience". *Local Environment*, 4(3):257–278.

Blatner, A. (2000). *Foundations of psychodrama.* New York: Springer Publishing Company.

Bourdieu, P. (1977). *Outline of a theory of practice.* Cambridge: Cambridge University Press

Bourdieu, P. (1990). *The logic of practice.* Cambridge: Polity Press.

Brockett, O. G. and Ball, R. J. (2004). *The essential theatre.* 8th Edition. California: Wadsworth/Thomas Learning.

Brown, R. and Cehajic-Clancy, S. (2008). "Dealing with the past and facing the future: Mediators of the effect of collective guilt and shame in Bosnia and Herzogovina". https://doi.org/10.1002/ejsp.466. Retrieved 04/28/2018

Bruhn, J. G. (2005). *The sociology of community connections.* Boston, MA: Kluwer Academic/Plenum Publishers, New York.

Butler, J. (1993). *Bodies that matter: On the discursive limits of sex.* London: Routledge.

Butler, J. (2004). "Performative acts and gender constitution: An essay in phenomenology and feminist theory". In Henry Bial (Ed.) *The Performance Studies Reader*, pp. 154–166. New York: Routledge.

Carlson, M. (2004). *Performance: A critical introduction.* 2nd Edition New York: Routledge.

Carmichael, J., Tansey, J. and Robinson, J. (2004). "An integrated assessment modeling tool". *Global Environmental Change*, 14(2):171–183.

Carmichael, J., Talwar, S., Tansey, J. and Robinson, J. (2005). "Where do we want to be? Making sustainability indicators integrated, dynamic and participatory". In Rhonda Philips (Ed.) *Community indicators measuring systems.* pp.178–204.

Cerulo, K. A. (1997). "Identity construction : New issues, new directions". *Annual Review of Sociology* 1997 23:1, 385–409.

Chiang, M. M. (2008). "Research on music and healing in ethnomusicology and music therapy". Diss. University of Maryland.

Cohen-Cruz, J. (Ed.) (1998), *Radical street performance: An international anthology.* London: Routledge.

Cohen-Cruz, J. (2010), *Engaging performance: Theatre as call and response.* London: Routledge.

Cohen–Cruz, J. and Schutzman, M. (Ed.) (1994), *Playing boal: Theatre, therapy, activism.* London and New York: Routledge.

Coleman, S. and Crang, M. (2002). "Grounded tourists, travelling theory". In Simon Coleman and Mike Crang (Eds.) *Tourism: Between place and performance.* pp. 1–19. New York: Berghahn.

Conquergood, D. (2002). "Performance studies: Interventions and radical research". *TDR/The Drama Review,* 46(2): pp. 145–156.

Conquergood, D. (2006). "Rethinking ethnography: Towards a critical cultural politics". In D. Soyini Madison and Judith Hamera (Eds.) *The SAGE handbook of performance studies.* pp. 351–365. Thousand Oaks, CA: SAGE.

Cordula, R. and König, U. (2017). "Collective trauma and resilience: Key concepts in transforming war-related identities". In B. Austin and M. Fischer(Eds.) *Berghof handbook dialogue series* No. 11. Berlin: Berghof Foundation.

Coult, T. and Kershaw B. (1983). *Engineers of the imagination: The welfare state handbook.* London: Methuen.

Crouch, D. (2001). "Spatialities and the feeling of doing". *Social & Cultural Geography,* 2(1):61–75.

Crouch, D. (2003). "Spacing, performing, and becoming: Tangles in the mundane". *Environment and Planning,* A 35(11):1945–1960.

Federal Ministry of Information and Culture. (1988). *Cultural policy for Nigeria.* Lagos: Federal Government Press.

Cummins, S., Findlay, A., Higgins, C.(2008). "Reducing inequalities in health and diet: Findings from a study on the impact of a food retail development". *Environment and Planning* A, 40(2): 402–422.

Davies, C. A. (1998). *Reflexive ethnography: A guide for researching selves and others.* New York: Routledge.

Davies, D. (2004). *Art as performance.* Massachusetts: Blackwell Publishing.

de Certeau, M. (1984). *The practice of everyday life.* Berkeley: University of California Press.

de Graft, J. C. (1983). "Roots of African drama". *African literature today 8, Drama.* Vol. III.

Delgado, M. (2019). *Urban youth trauma: Using community intervention to overcome gun violence.* Maryland: Rowman and Littlefield.

Delormier, T., Frohlich, K. L. and Potvin, L. (2009). "Food and eating as social practice – understanding eating patterns as social phenomena and implications for public health". *Sociology of Health & Illness,* 31(2): 215–228.

Dewsbury, J. D. (2000). "Performativity and the event: enacting a philosophy of difference". *Environment and Planning* D 18(4):473–496.

Doki, G. A. (2006). *Traditional theatre in perspective: Signs and significations in Igbe, Girinya and Kwaghhir.* Makurdi: Aboki Publishers.

Dolan, J. (2005). *Utopia in performance.* Ann Arbor: University of Michigan Press.

Duxbury, N. and Jeannotte S. (Ed.) (2011). *Culture and Local Governance 3* (1–2).

Dwyer, K. (1999). *Moroccan dialogues: Anthropology in question.* Baltimore: John Hopkins.

Ezeifeka, C. (2019). "Us" versus "Them": Ethnic identity construction in Nigerian political discourse. *Journal of English Department NAU, 6*(3): 56–64. https://doi.org/10.30845/ijll.v6n3p8.

Fearnow, M. (2007). *Theatre and the good: The value of collaborative play.* Youngstown, NY: Cambria Press.

Fischer-Lichte, E. (2014). "Culture as performance: Theatre history as cultural history". ACTAS/Proceedings, http://ww3.fl.ul.pt/centros_invst/teatro/pagina/Publicaoes/Actas/erika_def.pdf (Accessed April 28, 2014).

Fischer-Lichte, E. (2014). *The Routledge introduction to theatre and performance studies.* London: Routledge.

Fischer-Lichte, E. (2014). *Theatre and performance studies.* London: Routledge.

Fischer-Lichte, E. and Saskya, I. J. (2008). *The transformative power of performance.* Abingdon, Oxon: Routledge.

Frohlich, K. L., Corin, E. and Potvin, L. (2001). "A theoretical proposal for the relationship between context and disease". *Sociology of Health & Illness, 23*(6): 776–797.

Fulani, I. D. (2017, July 17). Poor funding affecting Nigeria's Great Green Wall Project. Premium Times. Retrieved from http://www.premiumtimesng.com/regional/nnorth-east/237217-poor-funding-affecting-nigerias-great-green-wallproject.html. Retrieved 06/10/2018

Gibson, J. J. (1979). *The ecological approach to visual perception.* Boston: Houghton Mifflin Company.

Giddens, A. (1986). *The constitution of society: Outline of the theory of structuration.* Berkeley and Los Angeles: University of California Press.

Goffman, E. (1959). *The presentation of self in everyday life.* New York: Doubleday.

Goffman, E. (1968). *Asylums.* London: Penguin Books.

Goodill, S. W. (2006). "Dance/movement therapy for people living with medical illness". In: S. C. Koch and I. Bräuninger (Eds.)*Advances in dance/movement therapy: Theoretical perspectives and empirical findings.* Berlin: Logos.

Haedicke, S. D. and Nellhaus, T. (2001). *Performing democracy: International perspectives on urban community-based performances.* Ann Arbor: University of Michigan Press.

Hall, S. and Jefferson, T. (Ed.) (1993), *Resistance through rituals: Youth subcultures in post-war Britain.* London: Routledge.

Hammersley, M. and Atkinson, P. (1983). *Ethnography: Principles in practice.* London: Tavistock.

Haraway, D. (1988). "Situated knowledges: The science question in feminism and the privilege of partial perspective". *Feminist Studies,* 14(3):575–599.

Hargreaves, T. (2011). "Practice-ing behaviour change: Applying social practice theory to pro-environmental behaviour change". *Journal of Consumer Culture,* 11(1):79–99. Retrieved April 15, 2012.

Harrison, P. (2000). "Making sense: Embodiment and the sensibilities of the everyday". *Environment and Planning D: Society and Space,* 18:497–517.

Hastrup, K. (2007). "Performing the world: Agency, anticipation and creativity". In Elizabeth Hallam and Tim Ingold (Eds.) *Creativity and cultural improvisation.* pp. 193–206. Oxford: Berg.

Hawkes, J. (2001). *The fourth pillar of sustainability: Culture's essential role in public planning.* IL: Common Ground.

Hawkes, J. (2002). "Creative engagement". *Artwork Magazine,* December, 10–15.

Hetherington, K. (2003). "Spatial textures: Place, touch, and praesentia". *Environment and Planning A* 35(11):1933–1944.

Hilton, J. (1987). *Performance.* London: Macmillan.

Hines, J.,Hungerford, H. and Tomera, A. (1986). "Analysis and synthesis of research on responsible environmental behaviour: A meta analysis". *Journal of Environmental Education,* 18(2):1–8.

Hirschberger, G. (2018). "Collective trauma and the social construction of meaning". *Front Pschol.* Published 2018 Aug 10. DOI:10.3389/fpsyg.2018.01441.

Holland, D., Lachicotte, W. Jr., Skinner, D., & Cain, C. (2001). *Identity and agency in cultural worlds.* New Edition. Cambridge, MA: Harvard University Press.

Horn, A. (1981). "Ritual, drama and the theatrical: The case of Bori spirit mediumship". InY. Ogunbiyi(Ed.)*Drama and theatre in Nigeria: A Critical Profile.* pp.184–202. Lagos: Nigerian Magazine.

Horne, R. E., Maller, C. J. and Lane, R. (2011). "Remaking home: The reuse of goods and materials in Australian households". In R. Lane and A. Gorman-Murray (Eds.) *Material geographies of household sustainability.* pp.89–111. Surrey, United Kingdom: Ashgate.

Horton, D. (2003). "Green distinctions: The performance of identity among environmental activists".In Bronislaw Szerszynski, Wallace Heim and Claire Waterton (Eds.) *Nature performed: Environment, culture and performance*. pp. 63–77. Oxford: Blackwell.

Huizinga, J. (2004). "The nature and significance of play as a cultural phenomenon". In Henry Bial (Ed.) *The performance studies reader*. pp. 117–120. New York: Routledge.

Illa, J. E. (1982). "Wole Soyinka: Some philosophical questions". A seminar paper delivered at Ahmadu Bello University, Zaria.

Imhoff, R., Bilewicz, M. and Erb, H. (2012). "Collective regret and collective guilt: Different emotional reactions to historical atrocities". *European Journal of Social* Psychology. Vol. 42 Issue 6. Pp. 729-742

Ingold, T. (2011). *Being alive: Essays on movement, knowledge and description.* New York, NY: Routledge.

International Crisis Group. (2017, September 19). Herders against Farmers: Nigeria's Expanding Deadly Conflict. *International Crisis Group Africa Report* (No. 252), 10. https://d2071andvip0wj.cloudfront.net/252-nigerias-spreadingherder-farmer-conflict.pdf. Retrieved 04/05/2019

Itulua-Abumere, F. (2014). "Sociological concepts of culture and identity". *www.Flourishabumere.Com*, (January), 1–5.

Jain, A. K. (2005). "Space and imagination". *International review of sociology, 15*(3), 529–545. https://doi.org/10.1080/03906700500272533. Retrieved 27/11/2018

Jeannotte, M. S. (2016). Story-telling about place: Engaging citizens in cultural mapping. *City, Culture and Society, 7*(1). https://doi.org/10.1016/j.ccs.2015.07.004.

Johnson, M. (2008). *The meaning of the body: Aesthetics of human understanding.* Chicago: University of Chicago Press.

Kagan, S. (2011). *Art and sustainability: Connecting patterns for a culture of complexity.* Bielefeld: Transcript Verlag.

Kelman, H. C. (1973). "Violence without moral restraint: Reflections on the dehumanization of victims and victimizers". *Journal of Social Issues, 29*(4), 25–61

Kershaw, B. (1992), *The politics of performance: Radical theatre as cultural intervention.* London: Routledge.

Kershaw, B. (Ed.) (2004), *Cambridge history of British theatre: Volume III: Since 1895.* Cambridge: Cambridge University Press.

Khan, N. (1980). "The public-going theatre: Community and 'ethic' theatre". In S. Craig (Ed.)*Dreams and deconstructions: Alternative theatre in Britain*. Amber Lane: Ambergate.

Klein, A. (1989). *The healing power of humor*. Los Angeles, CA: Jeremy P. Tarker, Inc.

Kollmuss, A. and AgyemanJ. (2002). "Mind the gap: Why do people act environmentally and what are the barriers to pro-environmental behaviour?" *Environmental Education Research*, 8(3):239–260.

Kriesberg, L. (1989). *Intractable conflicts and their transformations*. New York: Syracuse University.

Kuppers, P. (2007). *Community performance: An introduction*. London & New York: Routledge.

Kuppers, P. and Robertson, G. (2007). *The community performance reader*. London: Routledge.

Kwaja, A. M. C. (2013, March 13). Trends and patterns of violence and insecurity in Plateau State, Presentation at the Peace Architecture Dialogue (PAD). *Search for Common Ground*.

Kwaja, A. M. C. (2013, April 1). In search of humanitarian action plan: Combating desertification in the Sahel region of West Africa. Searchlight. Retrieved from https://futurechallenges.org/local/searchlight/in-search-ofhumanitarian-action-plan-combating-desertification-in-the-sahel-region-of-west-africa/. Retrieved 06/07/2019

Kwaja, A. M. C. (2014). Blood, cattle and cash: Cattle rustling and Nigeria's bourgeoning underground economy. *West Africa Insight*,4 (3).

Federal Government of Nigeria, (1978). Land Use Decree No.6, Cap 202. Laws of the Federation of Nigeria.

LeCompte, M. D. and Schensul, J. J. (1999a). *Analysing and interpreting ethnographic data:ethnographer's toolkit 5*. London: Altamira Press

LeCompte, M. D. and Schensul, J. J. (1999b). *Designing and conducting ethnographic research: Ethnographer's toolkit 1*. London: Altamira Press.

Levi, H. (2005). "Reflexivity". In Horowitz Maryanne Cline (Ed.)*New dictionary of the history of ideas, Vol. 5: Physics to Syncretism*. Detroit: Charles Scribner's Sons.

Littlejohn, S. W. and Foss, K. A. (2009). *Encyclopedia of communication theory*. Vol. 1 Thousand Oaks, CA: SAGE Publications.

Martin, R. (1997). "Dance ethnography and the limits of representation". In *Meaning in motion: New cultural studies of dance*. pp. 321–344. Durham: Duke University Press.

May, T. (2011). "'This is my neighbourhood!' - Community identity, ideology and performance".

Mbachaga, D. J. and Ukuma, S. T. (2012). "Cultural ethos in traditional African performances: The Tiv *Nyamtswam* in perspective". In S. E. Ododo(Ed.) *Fireworks for a Lighting Aesthetician: Essays and Tributes in Honour of Duro Oni @ 60*. pp. 628–640. Lagos: CBAAC.

McConachie, B. (1998). "Approaching the 'structure of feeling' in grassroots theatre", *Theatre Topics*, 8(1), 33–53.

Mercy Corps. (2015). The Economic Costs of Conflict and the Benefits of Peace: Effects of Farmers-Pastoralist Conflict in Nigeria's Middle Belt on State, Sector, and National Economies. *Mercy Corps*. Retrieved from https:// www. mercycorps.org/sites/default/files/Mercy%20Corps%20Nigeria%20 State%20Costs%20of%20Conflict%20Policy%20 Brief%20July%202015.pdf Retrieved 01/03/2018

Moreno, J. L. (1956). *Sociometry and the science of man*. New York: Beacon House.

Moreno, J. L. Zerka and Jonathan (1964). *The first psychodramatic family*. New York: Beacon House Inc.

Myerhoff, B. (1986). "'Life not death in venice': Its second life" In Victor W. Turnerand Edward M. Bruner(Eds.) *The anthropology of experience*. pp. 261–288. Chicago: University of Illinois Press.

Myerhoff, B. and Ruby, J. (Eds.) (1982). *The cracked mirror: Reflexive perspectives in anthropology*. Philadelphia: University of Pennsylvania Press.

Newton, D. (2014). "Performativity and the performer-audience relationships: Shifting perspectives and collapsing binaries". *The SOAS Journal of Postgraduate Research 7*, pp. 3–13.

Nicholson, H. (2005a). *Applied drama: The gift of theatre*. Macmillan, Hampshire and New York: Palgrave.

Nwoko, D. (1981). "Search for a New African Theatre". In Y. Ogunbiyi(Ed.)*Drama and theatre in Nigeria: A critical source book*. Lagos: Nigerian Magazine.

Nzekwu, O. (1981). Masquerade. In Ogunbiyi, Y. (Ed.)*Drama and theatre in Nigeria: A critical profile*. pp. 131–135. Lagos: Nigerian Magazine.

Nzewi, M. (1978). "Traditional African theatre from a sociological perspective". *The arts and civilization of black and African perspectives*. Vol.1. Lagos: Centre for Black and African Arts and Civilizations.

Nzewi, M. (1979). "Traditional theatre practice". In *Nigerian magazine*. pp.128–129.

Obaje, U. G. (2010). "Resolving Nigeria's leadership crises via traditional performances: The example of Aboga masquerade". InE. Dandauraand

A. Asigbo(Eds.)*Theatre, culture and re-imaging Nigeria*. pp. 292–302. Keffi: SONTA.

Ododo, S. E. (2015). *Facekuerade theatre: A performance model from Ebira- Ekue-chi*. Maiduguri: SONTA.

Ogunba, O. (1979). "Traditional African festival drama". In O. Ogunbaand A. Irele(Eds.) *Theatre in Africa*. Ibadan: University Press.

Ogunbiyi, Y. (1981). *Drama and theatre in Nigeria: A critical source book*. Lagos: Nigerian Magazine.

Okpewho, I. (Ed.)(1990). *The oral performance in Africa*. Ibadan: Spectrum Books.

Orngu, C. S., Ikpanor, E. T. and Kertyo, P. M. (Eds.) (2019). *Tiv Displacements in Benue, Nasarawa and Taraba States, 2013–2019*. (Commissioned by Msugh Moses Kembe, Vice Chancellor, Benue State University, Makurdi). Makurdi: BSU Press.

Osayin, B. (1988). "The concept of African total theatre and its implications for African unity". In ZaccheusAli(Ed.) *African unity: The cultural foundations*. pp. 153–162. S. Lagos: CBAAC.

Owens, S. (2000). "'Engaging the public': information and deliberation in environmental policy". *Environment and Planning A* 32:1141–1148.

Owens, S. and Driffill, L. (2008). "How to change attitudes and behaviours in the context of energy". *Energy Policy, 36* (12):4412–4418.

Ozumba, G. O. (1997). "A resume of Aquinas's philosophical thought". In Godfrey O. Ozumba (Ed.) *The great philosophers*. Vol. ii, Aba: Vitalis Books.

Ozumba, G. O. and Alabi, S. Y. (Eds.) (2002). *Landmarks in aesthetics studies*. Makurdi: Microtreachers and Associates.

Pavlicevic, M. and Ansdell, G. (2004) (eds.) *Community music therapy*. London: Jessica Kingsley Publishers.

Payne, H. (1992). *Dance movement therapy: Theory and practice*. London: Routledge.

Phelan, P. (1993). *Unmarked: The politics of performance*. London: Routledge.

Phelan, P. and Lane, J. (1998). *The ends of performance*. New York: New York University Press.

Portolés, J. B. and Šešić, M. D. (2017). "Cultural rights and their contribution to sustainable development: Implications for cultural policy". *International Journal of Cultural Policy*. 23 (2): 159–173.

Reckwitz, A. (2002). "Toward a theory of social practices: A development in culturalist theorizing". *European Journal of Social Theory*. 5(2): 243–263.

Riggs, A. (2010). "The creative space: Art and wellbeing in the shadow of trauma, grief and loss". PhD Thesis, Victoria University.

Robinson, J. (2003). "Future subjunctive: Backcasting as social learning". *Futures* 35(8):839–856.

Robinson, J. (2004). "Squaring the circle? Some thoughts on the idea of sustainable development". *Ecological Economics* 48(4):369–384.

Robinson, J. (2008). "Being undisciplined: Transgressions and intersections in academia and beyond". *Futures* 40(1):70–86.

Robinson, J. and Tansey, J. (2006). "Co-production, emergent properties and strong interactive social research: The Georgia Basin Futures Project". *Science and Public Policy* 33(2):151–160.

Robinson, J. and Tinker, J. (1997). "Reconciling ecological, economic, and social imperatives: A new conceptual framework". In Surviving Globalism: Social and Environmental Dimensions. pp. 71–94. London ; New York: Macmillan ; St. Martin's Press.

Robinson, J., , Carmichael, J. VanWynsberghe, R., Journaey, M., and Larson, R. (2006). "Sustainability as a problem of design: Interactive science in the Georgia Basin". *Integrated Assessment* 6(4):165–192.

Robinson, J., Burch, S., Talwar, S., O'Shea, M., and Walsh, M. (2011). "Envisioning sustainability: Recent progress in the use of participatory backcasting approaches for sustainability research". Technological Forecasting and Social Change.

Román, D. (1998). *Acts of intervention: Performance, gay culture, and AIDS.* Bloomington: Indiana University Press.

Rothenbuhler, E. W. (1998). *Ritual communication: From everyday conversation to mediated ceremony.* London: SAGE.

Ruud, E. (1998). *Music therapy: Improvisation, communication and culture.* Gilsum NH: Barcelona Publishers.

Schatzki, T. (1996). *Social practices: A Wittgensteinian approach to human activity and the social.* Cambridge: Cambridge University Press.

Schatzki, T. R. (2001). *Social practices.* Cambridge, UK: Cambridge University Press.

Schatzki, T. R. (2002). *The site of the social: A philosophical account of social life and change.* University Park, Pennsylvania: Penn State University Press.

Schechner, R. (1985). *Between theatre and anthropology.* Philadelphia: University of Pennsylvania Press.

Schechner, R. (1993). *The future of ritual: Writings on culture and performance.* New York: Routledge.

Schechner, R. (1998). "What is performance studies anyway?" In Peggy Phelan and Jill Lane (Eds.) *The Ends of Performance*, pp. 357–362. New York, NY: New York University Press.

Schechner, R. (2002). *Performance studies: An introduction*. London: Routledge.

Schinina, G. (2004). "Here we are: Social theatre and some open questions about its developments". *TDR: The Drama Review*, 48.

Schneider, W. and Gad, D. (2014). *Good governance for cultural policy: An African-European research about arts and development*. Frankfurt: Peter Lang

Schutzman, M. (2006). "Ambulant pedagogy". In D. Soyini Madison and Judith Hamera (Eds.) *The SAGE handbook of performance studies*. pp. 278–295. Thousand Oaks, CA: SAGE.

Shove, E. (2003). *Comfort, cleanliness and convenience - The social organization of normality*. Oxford: Berg.

Shove, E. (2010). "Beyond the ABC: Climate change policy and theories of social change". *Environment and Planning A* 42: 1272–1285.

Shove, E. (2010). "Beyond the ABC: Climate change policy and theories of social change". *Environment and Planning A* 42(6):1273–1285.

Shove, E. and Pantzar, M. (2005). "Consumers, producers and practices". *Journal of consumer culture* 5(1):43–64.

Shove, E. and Pantzar, M. (2007). "Recruitment and reproduction: The careers of and carriers of digital photography and floorball". *Human Affairs* 17: 154–167.

Shove, E. and Walker, G. (2010). "Governing transitions in the sustainability of everyday life". *Research Policy* 39(4):471–476.

Shove, E., Pantzar, M. and Watson, M. (2012). *The dynamics of social practice: Everyday life and how it changes*. London, UK: SAGE.

Shove, E., Watson, M., Hand, M. and Ingram, J. (2007). *The design of everyday life*. Oxford: Berg.

Shusterman, R. (2005). "The silent, limping body of philosophy". In T. Carmen and N. Hansen (Eds.) *The Cambridge Companion to Merleau-Ponty*. pp. 151–180. Cambridge: Cambridge University Press.

Silverman, M. J. (2003). "The influence of music on the symptoms of psychosis: A meta-analysis". *Journal of Music Therapy* 40(1): 27–40.

Skjoldager-nielsen, K. and Edelman, J. (2014). *Liminality*, 7:1–6.

Stige, B. (2002). *Culture-centred music therapy*. Gilsum, NH: Barcelona Publishers.

Strengers, Y. and Maller, C. (2011). "Integrating health, housing and energy policies: social practices of cooling". *Building Research & Information* 39(2): 1–15.

Tansey, J., Robinson, J., , Carmichael, J., and VanWynsberghe, R.(2002). "The future is not what it used to be: Participatory integrated assessment in the Georgia Basin". *Global Environmental Change* 12(2):97–104.

The Peace and Security Forum. (2017). Resolving the herders/farmers conflict in Nigeria, Policy Brief.

Thrift, N. (1996). *Spatial formations*. London: SAGE Publications.

Thrift, N. (1999a). "Entanglements of power: shadows?" In J. Sharp, P. Routledge, C. Philo and R. Paddison (Eds.)*Geographies of Domination/Resistance*. pp. 269–277. London: Routledge.

Thrift, N. (1999b). "Steps to an ecology of place". In Doreen Massey, John Allen and Philip Sarre (Eds.) *Human Geography Today*. pp. 295–322. Cambridge, UK: Polity Press.

Thrift, N. (2000a). "Afterwords". *Environment and Planning D: Society and Space* 18(2):213–255.

Thrift, N. (2000b). "Dead or Alive?" InI. Cook, D. Crouch, S. Naylor, and J. Ryan. *Cultural Turns*. pp. 1–6. Harlow, Essex: Prentice-Hall.

Thrift, N. (2004). "Driving in the City". *Theory, Culture & Society* 21:41–59.

Thrift, N. and Dewsbury, J. D. (2000). "Dead geographies and how to make them live". *Environment and Planning D: Society and Space* 18:411–432.

Throsby, D. (1995). "Culture, economics and sustainability". *Journal of Cultural Economics* 19(3):199–206.

Throsby, D. (2017). "Culturally sustainable development: Theoretical concept or practical policy instrument?" *International Journal of Cultural Policy*, 23(2), 133–147.

Tuan, Y. (2001). *Space and place: the perspective of experience*. Minnesota: University of Minnesota Press.

Turner, V. (1967). "Betwixt and between: The liminal period in Rites de Passage". In V. Turner and V. W. Turner *The forest of symbols*. Ithaca, NY: Cornell University Press.

Turner, V. (1974), *Dramas, fields and metaphors: Symbolic action in human society*. Ithaca, NY: Cornell University Press.

Turner, V. (1977). "Liminality and Communitas: Form and attributes of rites of passage". *The Ritual Process. Structure and Anti-Structure*, 96–130. Retrieved from http://www.iupui.edu/~womrel/Rel433 Readings/Turner_Liminality&Communitas.pdf. 22/04/2018

Turner, V. (1980). "Social dramas and stories about them". *Critical inquiry* 7(1):141–168.

Turner, V. (1982). *From ritual to theatre: The human seriousness of play*. New York: Performing Arts Journal Publications.

Turner, V. (1988). *Anthropology of performance*. New York: PAJ Publications.

Turner, V. W. and Bruner, E. M. (Eds.) (1986). *The anthropology of experience*. Chicago: University of Illinois.

Ukuma, T. S. (2014). "Cultural aesthetics in Tiv traditional performances: A critical perspective". *African Journal of Local Societies Initiative*. 3:40–49.

van der Merwe, S. (2010). *The effect of dance and movement intervention program on the perceived emotional well-being of a clinical sample of adolescents*. Pretoria: University of Pretoria.

Van Erven, E. (2001). *Community theatre: Global perspectives*. London, New York: Routledge.

Vanwynsberghe, R., Carmichael, J. and Khan, S. (2007). "Conceptualizing sustainability: Simulating concrete possibilities in an imperfect world". *Local Environment* 12(3):279–293.

Volkan, V. D. (1997). *Bloodlines: From ethnic pride to ethnic terrorism*. New York: Farrar, Straus and Giroux.

Volkan, V. D. (2004). *Blind trust: Large groups and their leaders in times of crisis and terror*. Charlottesville, VA: Pitchstone Publishing.

Whatmore, S. (2006). "Materialist Returns: Practising cultural geography in and for a more-than-human world". *Cultural Geographies* 13(4):600–609.

Williams, G. H. (2003). "The determinants of health: structure, context and agency". *Sociology of Health & Illness* 25(3): 131–154.

Williams, R. (1976). *Keywords: A vocabulary of culture and society*. London: Fontana.

Williams, S. J. (1995). "Theorising class, health and lifestyles: Can Bourdieu help us?" *Sociology of Health & Illness* 17(5): 577–604.

Yinka, A. J. (1978). "Theatricalism and traditional African theatre". *The arts and civilization of Black and African perspectives*. Vol. 1. Lagos: Centre for Black and African Arts and Civilizations.

Young, I. M. (1990). "The ideal of community and the politics of difference". In L. Nicholson (Ed.)*Feminish/Postmodernism*. London: Routledge.

Zontou, Z. (2011). "Applied theatre and drugs: Community, creativity and hope". Thesis. University of Manchester.

Studien zur Kulturpolitik
Cultural Policy

Herausgegeben von / Edited by Prof. Dr. Wolfgang Schneider

Band 1 Robert Peise: Ein Kulturinstitut für Europa. Untersuchungen zur Institutionalisierung kultureller Zusammenarbeit. 2003.

Band 2 Angela Koch: Kommunale Kulturorganisation in den USA. Strukturen, Handlungsmuster, Interdependenzen. 2005.

Band 3 Sabine Dorscheid: Staatliche Kunstförderung in den Niederlanden nach 1945. Kulturpolitik versus Kunstautonomie. 2005.

Band 4 Dirk Meyer-Bosse: Geld-Geber. Die Bedeutung von Sparkassen für die Kulturförderung in Deutschland. 2005.

Band 5 Kai Reichel-Heldt: Filmfestivals in Deutschland. Zwischen kulturpolitischen Idealen und wirtschaftspolitischen Realitäten. 2007.

Band 6 Annette Wostrak: Kooperative Kulturpolitik. Strategien für ein Netzwerk zwischen Kultur und Politik in Berlin. 2008.

Band 7 Frank Sommer: Kulturpolitik als Bewährungsprobe für den deutschen Föderalismus. 2008.

Band 8 Sandra Soltau: Freie Musikszene – Perspektiven für ein innovatives Konzertwesen? 2010.

Band 9 Reiner Küppers: Künstlerinnen und Künstler zwischen kreativer Freiheit und sozialer Sicherheit. Ein Diskurs zur Kulturpolitik in Zeiten europäischer Integration. 2010.

Band 10 Anne-Kathrin Bräu: Corporate Citizenship in Regensburg. Unternehmenskommunikation als Kulturpolitik. 2011.

Band 11 Dieter Kramer: Von der Freizeitplanung zur Kulturpolitik. Eine Bilanzierung von Gewinnen und Verlusten. 2011.

Band 12 Joerg Schumacher: Das Ende der kulturellen Doppelrepräsentation. Die Auswärtige Kulturpolitik der Bundesrepublik Deutschland und der DDR am Beispiel ihrer Kulturinstitute 1989/90. 2011.

Band 13 Azadeh Sharifi: Theater für Alle? Partizipation von Postmigranten am Beispiel der Bühnen der Stadt Köln. 2011.

Band 14 Usa Beer: Zwischen Avantgarde und Auftrag. Bildende KünstlerInnen und ihre Kompetenzen als gesellschaftliches Potenzial. 2012.

Band 15 Jan Büchel: Fernsehen für Europa. Transnationale mediale Öffentlichkeit als kulturpolitischer Auftrag der EU. 2013.

Band 16 Wolfgang Schneider / Daniel Gad (eds.): Good Governance for Cultural Policy. An African-European Research about Arts and Development. 2014.

Band 17 Claudia Burkhard: Kulturpolitik als Strukturpolitik? Konzepte und Strategien deutscher und italienischer Kulturpolitik im Vergleich. 2015.

Band 18 Annika Holland: Kulturpolitik für kulturelle Vielfalt. Rezeption und Implementierung der UNESCO-Konvention zum Schutz und zur Förderung der Vielfalt kultureller Ausdrucksformen in Deutschland. 2016.

Band 19 Saskia Helene Jeanne Weiss: Europäischer Minderheitenschutz am nationalen Beispiel der Regionalsprachen in Frankreich. 2017.

Band   20   Christian Müller-Espey: Zukunftsfähigkeit gestalten. Untersuchung nachhaltiger Strukturen soziokultureller Zentren. 2019.

Band   21   Shadrach Teryila Ukuma: Cultural Performances. A Study on Managing Collective Trauma amongst Displaced Persons in Daudu, Benue State, Nigeria. 2021.

www.peterlang.com